Carpe diem

Carpe diem

Enjoying Every Day
with a Terminal Illness

Ed Madden

Jones and Bartlett Publishers
Boston   London

Editorial, Sales, and Customer Service Offices

Jones and Bartlett Publishers
One Exeter Plaza
Boston, MA 02116
617-859-3900
1-800-832-0034

Jones and Bartlett Publishers International
7 Melrose Terrace
London W6 7RL
England

Library of Congress Cataloging-in-Publication Data

Madden, Ed.
   Carpe diem : enjoying every day with a terminal illness / Ed Madden.
      p.   cm.
    ISBN 0-86720-782-5
    1. Madden, Ed—Health.   2. Multiple myeloma—Patients—United States—Biography.   3. Terminally ill—United States—Biography.
   I. Title.
   RC280.B6M335   1993
   362.1'9699'4—dc20
   [B]
                                                    93-12746
                                                        CIP

Cover design: Bruce Kennett
Interior design and production: John A. Servideo
Typesetting: Pure Imaging

Printed in the United States of America
97 96 95 94   10 9 8 7 6 5 4 3 2

To
Barbara Madden
and
Laura Madden
the two women
who share my home
and make this journey
of mine
a daily paradise

Preface

*I*n late June 1990, the several disorders that had been troubling me for over five months were explained by a simple diagnosis: cancer. My doctor outlined with a kindness and sadness that meant much to me, that multiple myeloma is not curable, but that with proper treatment, I should have a few years.

My reaction was action. I ran around notifying family and friends, decided on an oncologist, began radiation treatment and tried to keep working, despite some serious pain. Then I sat with Eddie Forry, the publisher of *The Reporter*, a local paper for which I had been writing a column. We both had already come to the same conclusion—that I should start writing a second column about my new journey.

The following pages are filled with most of the columns that I've written every two weeks over the past two and more years. Because they undoubtedly reveal change and growth that is not readily apparent to me, I've left them, with one exception, in the order they appeared.

Many people, those ailing, some caregivers and numerous friends, both old and new, have told me that the columns aided in their own journeys. I hope this collection will be a way of reaching out to others, to let them know they're not alone.

*A*cknowledgments

Although my name alone appears on the title page, this book and the columns that make up its parts were the work of many people.

Eddie Forry, publisher of *The Reporter*, has been involved in my columns from their earliest conceptualizing. His wife and partner, Mary Forry, played a role as typesetter and proofreader. They both played a far greater role as my friends.

Many of the staff at *The Reporter* played a part both in the columns and in the predecessor book that we published: Ginny Aveni, Denise Doherty, Barbara McDonough, and particularly the Mullen sisters, Peggy and Barbie, who are not only involved in my columns, but now, fortunately, in my life.

And then there is Sue Asci, about whom I cannot say enough. A friend for many years, my editor at *The Reporter* for a couple, she's given me more support on this journey than I can ever tell her.

Carpe diem

*T*he
Journey Begins

I have just entered upon a new adventure, the most exciting, challenging, spirited experience of all my 53 years. I've discovered I have cancer.

Of course, had I been given the choice of a weekend with Kathleen Turner, a sailing trip to Bermuda or cancer, the ailment would most definitely not have won out. But, as in so many of the other wonderful things that have happened to me — my birth, choice of parents and siblings, my rearing in Boston, my schooling, my magnificent body and looks, the choice was not mine.

Like the new obnoxious kid in class, the cancer is here to stay. I can hate it, fume against it, pout and sulk, but that hurts only me. Or I can put it in its place and go on about my business, and that's what I intend to do. In either case, of course, I still have the cancer. It will be a game, played over the next months or years, a game that eventually the cancer undoubtedly will win, but I will score the maximum number of goals in the meantime. And like any sporting event, it will be the playing that is the fun.

But just as Ireland engaged Italy in the recent quarter-finals of the World Soccer cup, knowing the outcome in advance, I will enter my game with gusto and play with all my heart. I'll use the best resources that medical science has to offer me, but I have something even better — my own will and desire and spirit. We still have only sketchy knowledge of the power of our minds to control our bodies, but we do know it is mighty.

Of course, I will be the winner too. It will be through the agency of this cancer that I will pass over the River Jordan to the Elysian Fields, where the peace and happiness never end. That the cancer will take me out is only a presumption. Just as before I received my diagnosis,

I know neither the time nor manner of my death. However, at the moment I'm not investing heavily in tickets to the arrival of the third millennium in 2001, though I'm not precluding my attendance either.

The vocabulary of my new adventure is interesting. I tell people of my cancer and I speak of my death, but no one else, at least in my company, seems able to say those words. It seems they should not be uttered in polite society. The terms tragedy, crisis and trouble are not applicable here, for my new condition (more accurately, my newly discovered condition, for the cancer has probably been my close companion for years) is none of those. Cancer and dying and death are natural phenomena, the latter two the property of all of us.

This is the reason I decided to go public with my illness; not because my cancer and my death, whenever it may occur, are great newsmaking events. Rather it is to assist others to whom the revelation of their cancers or other terminal illnesses has been devastating. It always helps to know that we have companions on a journey.

These will not be stories about dying, but on the contrary, about living. It is true that we are born to die, but we must live first. So I will share with you my celebration of life.

For all of the years I've been on this earth, I've had only a single day in which to do anything — today. Yesterday is the matter of history books and tomorrow never seems to arrive. So today, as I have done for almost 20,000 todays, I shall enjoy the day. Join me. Quintus Horatius Flaccus, the Roman poet whom we know familiarly as Horace, said it well: *Carpe diem*.

An
Incalculable Wealth

I've never made much money, and doing so was never a matter of overriding importance with me. But I've suddenly discovered I'm one of the wealthiest men in the world. So many people, men and women, who, on hearing of my cancer, have spoken those priceless words, "I love you, Ed." Trump's billions can't buy those words. I've been smothered in hugs and kisses.

I find that the little kindnesses I've been able to do for others, time and effort that cost me so little, were received as great gifts and I've been bankrolling a cache of gratitude I knew nothing about. It is found money, and a currency so helpful in my new journey.

One of the fortuitous turnings in my life brought me to my current career as a private detective. For a fee I solve clients' problems, but I've occasionally been able to use the same abilities and facilities for the good of friends, in cases where a bill or an offer to pay would have insulted us both. I'm being paid now in so much more than money. Now I am the debtor, and with no ability to repay. It is truly humbling.

Humility, never one of my strong points, is a virtue that is being forced upon me now. It was a back problem that alerted me to the presence of the cancer, and it continues to render me, at least for the moment, unable to carry anything heavy or do any physical labor at all. Having been proud of my independence all these years, I find it very difficult to have to accept the ministrations of others. So, kicking and screaming, I'll become a humble man, and be proud of it.

The offers to help, to do anything I need, have come not only from friends, but from scant acquaintances. Relatives completed in two weekends yard work that I had planned to spend the next year doing. I dare not drive at the moment as I'm on pain medication, but I have enough offers of rides to take me around the globe. I even received a message from a statuesque woman whom I barely know that my shoes are welcome under her bed anytime. I'm still mulling over that one. Why did she wait till now to tell me?

One of the first blessings my parents conferred upon me was six brothers and sisters and a second was a family atmosphere that bred such love that we are today each others' closest friends. It was this that inspired my wife and me to move back here from New York–New Jersey 17 years ago. It's a move we've never regretted and from my new perspective it was the best move I ever made. Their love, company and support is now my daily bread. And my wife's family is doing just as much for me.

So, as I wrote in an earlier column, my cancer is not a tragedy or a problem. On the contrary, it has proved to be the key that opened the vault where these unknown, not to mention undeserved, treasures lie. I experience more love, concern, compassion and care on a daily basis than I ever doled out in a year. I now realize that I am one of the richest people in the world.

*W*ho
Am I Now?

I am not a cancer patient!

I know that statement rather flies in the face of previous articles describing my new adventure with cancer. My point is that those of us who have cancer or other major and life threatening illnesses can sometimes let the ailment overwhelm us, so that we think of ourselves only in terms of the sickness. But we are all so much more than that.

My new knowledge of the presence of cancer in no way affects my status as a husband and father, a private detective, a journalist, a photographer, a lover and a friend, a reader of poetry and a gardener. I also am the owner of a house, a few cameras, a car, a five-speed bicycle, many tools and some cancer.

It is important to note that I own the cancer. It does not own me. Nor does it define me, any more than any of the above titles offers any all-encompassing description of me. I am no different from the person I was two months ago before I knew I had the cancer, or a few years ago before the first plasma cell developed in an oddball direction.

So who am I? I am simply Ed Madden, whatever that means. I am loved by a few, liked by many, disliked by some. I am Ed Madden, a very flawed human being — a bit more physically flawed now than I had realized — but still trying to improve a bit day by day. A realistic sense of our own selves, with an appreciation of our myriad weaknesses, helps us to face critical illnesses. It has long been an important cog of my personal philosophy, and one about which I have taught and written at length, that we are all imperfect, flawed and weak. It is the daily struggle to better ourselves physically, spiritually, intellectually, and emotionally that makes life interesting and challenging. The arrival of a serious illness, therefore, does not change our direction, but only heightens the adventure.

Acceptance of ourselves as imperfect shows illnesses as natural phenomena, as more in a long chain of flaws that mark our lives. And if we have been used to starting anew with each sunrise to better ourselves by fighting against all our imperfections, then we simply include the new ailments on our list of things to improve.

Theologians tell us that when we reach heaven we will have achieved a state of perfection. But perfection sounds dull. What will we do all day?

We All Need Loving

*B*ill R. and I have been friends for ten or a dozen years, but we had other earlier things in common. We both went to the old Boston College High School in the South End of Boston, though Bill was a few years ahead of me. He was an altar boy at the Immaculate Conception church, connected to the school, and we were both friendly with a lot of the same priests there.

Billy and I also contracted cancer at about the same time this year. We met the other day for the first time since either of us was diagnosed. He was in University Hospital for his final chemotherapy. I was an outpatient at the same place for radiation therapy. We had a lot to talk about.

During our lengthy conversation, Bill asked, "Have you noticed how people avoid you?" The question hung there for a bit. I certainly had; I couldn't have missed it. The look of recognition and the quick turn in the other direction. The sudden interest in a store window. Or the need to hurry past with a quick howdeedo. Friends have called other friends about me, but have been afraid to call me. Billy and I have had identical experiences with this.

Suddenly and somewhat painfully, we've become pariahs, akin to the lepers of centuries past. Cancer has the lowest respectability rating of all ailments. Heart diseases and orthopedic procedures rate at the top. We don't hesitate to ask someone about his triple bypass or the steel rod that was put in his leg. But cancer? We not only can't mention it to the patient, but in talking about it our voice drops to a whisper. "Ed Madden has cancer."

Many people are devastated when they learn they have a cancer. But much of the fear, revulsion and shame they feel is a factor not of the medical implications but of society's jaundiced view of the disease.

There are about 100 types of cancer. Some are totally curable and many others can be put into remission for years. Still others, like my own, can be slowed down for lengthy periods. It is no longer true that people who are told they have cancer must go home to die. Most of us still have a lot of living to do first.

There may be people with cancer who don't want to talk about it. There probably are. But I don't know any. When I get together with my friends, we talk about things that are of importance to us. Today, as my knowledge of my cancer is still in its early stages and I'm carefully navigating through radiation and the beginnings of chemotherapy, it's important to me and to my friends and I want to, have to, talk about it.

Several friends and acquaintances have been wonderfully gracious at meeting me, asking gently how I am. The words come out more solicitously than the casual "How're ya doing?" leaving the opening gambit to me, giving me the option of mentioning my cancer or not. I have appreciated their kindness.

This is not an attempt to lay a guilt trip on friends who have been reluctant to talk to me. I know how hard it is. I was in their shoes too.

The day our doctors told Bill and me that we had cancer we were jolted. Getting cancer — or more correctly knowing that we have it — is a very painful experience. It is a time when, probably more than at any other time in our lives, we need our friends around us. We need to know we have friends. We need to celebrate that we are still among the living. We need to be loved.

Learning from the Mind

*L*ast year I wrote at different times and in another column about mind control and hypnosis. Now that I have cancer I need to learn much more about how the mind can control the body, diminish pain and even extend life.

Just the other day a friend was commenting on how her mother was told several years ago that she had leukemia, so "she went home, got into bed, faced the wall and died." Conversely, and more importantly, there are countless stories of people who were told they had little time to live, but they decided differently and prospered for years.

Many people have psychosomatic illnesses — sickness brought on by the mind. It is easy to understand how such ailments are cured by mental processes. But how are real bodily malfunctions reversed by brain power? This question arose for me just a few days after I had been diagnosed as having cancer. I visited a woman who has had my cancer, multiple myeloma, for six years. She looked perfectly healthy and functions as a school principal, never missing a day of work. It was a very positive experience for me and I felt buoyed. A few hours later when I was entertaining company at home I realized that the constant back pain that had announced the presence of my cancer was absent for the first time in over a month. I remained free of pain for some hours.

A couple of weeks later, also after a very happy experience, the back pain again vanished for several hours. Why? How? My own past experiments with self-hypnosis have enabled me to banish headaches, tiredness, and lassitude. If I were more skilled at hypnosis could I eliminate the back pain entirely? Could I reverse the course of the cancer itself?

In an attempt to answer some of these questions, I lunched last week with an old friend, Pat Brady, who is a hypnotherapist at

Marina Bay in Quincy, Mass. Pat regularly aids clients in quitting smoking, losing weight and improving their motivation and self image.

Pat, who operated the Boston Police Department's hypnosis unit until his retirement earlier this year, has been a student and practitioner of hypnosis for more than a decade, but still remains in awe of the mysterious power of the mind to affect the entire person.

"We are who we think we are," he commented the other day, following with "If you think you can or you think you can't, you're right."

During lunch and afterwards, Pat cited numerous cases of people who achieved goals, including improving their health, simply because they were determined to do so. Can a positive mindset improve or cure cancer? He's seen too much to set any limits on the power of the mind to accomplish any goals, but at the same time he cautioned that there are no guarantees.

Pat is a friend and colleague of the guru in the field of mind controlling our destinies — Bernie Siegel — a New Haven surgeon. His several books and tapes are a must for anyone wanting to dominate and change bodily functions via brain power. Siegel's tapes assist self hypnosis but it helps if the person has been guided through hypnosis first by an expert.

Just a day after meeting with Pat, I received a letter from a reader who was diagnosed six months ago with incurable cancer but was "given no concrete sense of what I could do about it except take my medicine." But a few weeks ago he was given Siegel's book, *Love, Medicine & Miracles*. The reader continued, "Siegel's point is that one's mind can control the immune system, and has caused not only remission, but cures in cases written off as hopeless by conventional medical thinking. In reading the book, I decided the shoe fit, and fully intend to be a survivor."

This is a new area of experimentation, and data are few. It doesn't matter that we can't say how or why it works. For those of us in good and poor health alike, it only matters that it does work. And no one can do it for us.

Death,
a Result of Birth

*L*ife threatening illnesses force us to look into the face of death. Those of us who learn we have cancer, people who have serious heart attacks, accident victims, we all find ourselves thinking of death no longer as an abstraction but as something that is happening to us.

Suddenly we speak of death in the first person rather than as the property of someone else. The obituary page now possesses a closeness. A wake or a funeral are premonitions, rather than just an opportunity to pray for a friend.

We must strike a balance here. Many of us with serious illnesses have a long time to live. Still, we have to accept the inevitable fact that death does hover closely for us and that the disease we know will probably be the agent of our deaths. But we also have to remember that today every person in the world is one day closer to death, whether or not they have a diagnosis of cancer or other life-threatening ailments. Many who are in perfect health today will precede us. No one will get out of this world alive.

The attitude with which we view death during our lives affects how we will approach it as it draws near. The images of death as skeletons, a dark figure with a scythe or as Charon poling his boat across the river Styx do us no favors. Death is part of a natural process that begins at the moment of our conceptions.

Some of us, facing death, grow angry and ask "Why me?" "Why do I have to die while the homeless bum on the corner, who is of no use to anyone, even himself, survives?" Anger can be both a positive and a negative drive, but I think in this instance it is misplaced. Death is simply a natural result of being born. We might more justly rail at our births than at our deaths.

I love to garden. Each spring as I take tiny seeds from their envelopes and place them in the soil, I marvel at the complexity and beauty of the process. Small and simple looking as they are, the seeds contain all the information and genes to produce a wonderful tomato or a beautiful zinnia. But in the process the seed itself dies. So too, the process of the constant renewal of this world, its ever present youth, demand that we come, do our thing and die.

I always thought that I would follow Madden family tradition and go out from a quick heart attack — and of course I still may. But we who are alerted to our deaths have the advantage of reconciling where it is needed, of healing wounds, so that those we leave behind will not suffer more than necessary at our passing.

I have found that facing death as I have these past few months has enabled me and those closest to me to deepen our love more than I could have imagined. This is a benefit of inestimable value and one that has made my sufferings well worth the price.

Facing the Door without Fear

*I*n the last column we walked to the door of death. This column is not usually dedicated to theological reflection, but since most of the readers of *The Reporter* are grounded in Judeo-Christian beliefs, I think that we have to pass through that portal and discuss my thoughts about what is on the other side.

I went to Catholic grade school and high school and learned to fear God. I came to know a God who was always watching me, who knew my innermost thoughts even before I did and who would have no hesitation about punishing me for the least transgression of his innumerable laws, or even more importantly, the rules of the church.

Following graduation from high school I had the good fortune to enter the Society of Jesus — the Jesuit order — where I made my home for the next dozen years. During those years I read, studied, learned, absorbed and prayed over the Old and New Testaments, the source of most of our knowledge of God and his dealings with his people.

I learned of a God who loved, and like any lover, was always ready to forgive. I studied a Jesus, the Messiah, the Christ, who taught mercy, compassion, and above all, love. I found that the image of God with which I had been imbued in my younger days was not the image that God himself had sought to portray in the Scriptures. I write this, not to cast any blame on my early teachers, but to show where I am now, and possibly to inspire some readers who are still living in dread fear of God to pick up their Bibles and read.

Those of us with terminal illnesses know that in a longer or shorter period we will be face to face with our God. I am not afraid. Jesus taught us to call God "Father." If we are more comfortable with the term, we could use "Mother" as well. Who loves more than a parent loves a child? Should I believe that my love for my daughter, which I consider boundless, is greater than God's love for me? If so, I would be a better parent than God.

No, my acceptance by God will depend not so much on how good or bad I've been here, but on how much he loves me. He loves me not because I am so loveable but because he is so loving. My sinfulness cannot discourage me when I read Jesus saying that it was for us sinners that he came. Some of the most tender moments in all the Gospels are the stories of his dealings with sinners. Never once did he condemn common sinners. Indeed he reserved his scorn for those who considered themselves righteous and law-abiding.

The Psalms bid us: "Bless Yahweh, my soul, and remember all his kindnesses in forgiving all your offenses...." It's been 3000 years since that was written. God's done a lot of pardoning in that time.

Our God is a God of love, of forgiveness, of mercy. Our God is a father and mother. This is the God of the Scriptures; this is the God that Jesus described to us. This is the God I've come to know these many latter years. This is the God who will welcome all us prodigal children back home soon.

Progressing without a Guide

We have no trouble learning how to get healthy, stay healthy and what to do with our good health. Daily papers, weekly and monthly magazines, endless televisions shows all dote on health.

But few writers tell us how to be sick. Yet virtually every man born to woman, and every woman too, spends days, weeks, months and even years, ailing. Where are the instructions? Where are the videos that show us how?

Several years ago an old friend of mine, Father Joe O'Kane, a veteran of years of teaching in Baghdad, was confined with cancer at Campion Center, the Jesuit infirmary in Weston, some 20 miles outside Boston. One day he said with a smile to one of his nurses, "Please let me know if I'm making any mistakes." Puzzled, she replied, "What do you mean, Father? What kind of mistakes?" "Well," Joe said, "I've never died before. I'm not sure I know how to do it right."

Writers like Dr. Bernie Siegal, in his *Love, Medicine & Miracles*, help us to have a positive attitude toward our ailments. An upbeat frame of mind can assist us in beating back many ills. But we must accept the fact that some diseases are with us to stay and that death will eventually come to us all.

It is now just four months since I found that I have an incurable cancer. Therefore, I have reached the end of my life. The end, in my case, may last for several years. Long time or short, this period imposes new duties and offers different challenges.

Prime among the duties is the preparation of my closest friends for my death. There is obviously nothing I can do to spare them the grief they will feel at my passing. But I can leave them with the best of memories. I can fill these days with happiness and joy and share with them the peace I feel in my new role. All the better if my death is still many years away. We'll all have, if you'll pardon the expression, a hell of a good time. This threat of death, then, is really providing a lesson in how to live.

We could, of course, make ourselves so disagreeable that the world will be glad to be rid of us. I heard a story just the other day about a woman whose abusive husband died suddenly. On getting the news, her only reaction was, "Thank God. I'm finally free of the s.o.b." I don't see that course of action as acceptable, however.

The challenges of this period are new. During times of suffering just keeping a smile on our faces can be a chore. Remembering to be grateful to our caregivers is important. But during times of improved health, we must each reach for goals that are suitable for our conditions. Reading, writing, visiting, traveling, learning still beckon. We must not stop living until we draw our final breath. In my case, this series of columns has presented itself as a major challenge and opportunity for me. What I write here these days I could never have penned earlier, lacking the experience of sickness and a terminal illness.

We can often draw much peace from dropping certain other goals that had preoccupied us until now. Raising a family, building a business, furthering a career are aims that have demanded the most energy from us. Now we who approach death can rest in the knowledge that we have done what we can and we must leave these cares in the hands of God. Peace!

Cancer
Therapies Vary

*T*here is perhaps only one thing more frightening to people than cancer and that is the treatments for cancer, specifically the most common: surgery, radiation and chemotherapy.

It may be that the great fear that surrounds the whole notion of cancer causes patients and their loved ones to be afraid of anything associated with the disease. Also, there are sometimes very difficult side effects of these treatments.

However, those of us affected with cancer know the disease won't go away on its own, and in most cases it will make progress unless we do something about it, so we, together with our doctors, have to make some decisions.

Surgery is called for in many cases, both as a diagnostic tool and as a corrective measure. Often the most sophisticated tests are unable to determine the ailment, so doctors must take an actual look. Some cancers can be cut out and for some lucky patients, this constitutes the cure.

In other instances the cancer is removed but the medical staff wants further treatment to ensure that none of the tumor cells remain. This then calls for radiation and/or chemotherapy. These two methods are sometimes used alone or in conjunction, without surgery, to shrink and eliminate tumors.

Radiation is something we get every time we go out into the sun. We also get it every time we have an X-ray. The radiation we receive for cancer is generally X-ray or electron rays. These rays are directed to the cancerous tumor, passing in many instances through skin, flesh and bone to reach the growth. The rays have the ability to kill the cancerous cells, sometimes shrinking the cancer to nothing.

There may be problems associated with radiation. Just as too many of the sun's rays can cause burning of the skin, so these rays can cause burns, sometimes on the skin, other times of interior tissue and organs. It is the burning of organs that can cause reactions such as vomiting.

Chemotherapy seems to cause the most confusion, if not the most problems. The word "chemo" is the root of the word chemical, and means just that — a chemical therapy, a medicine. Every time we take an aspirin for a headache, we are giving ourselves chemotherapy, though we usually reserve that term only for cancer therapy.

There are over 50 drugs that are commonly used to battle cancer, either alone or, frequently, in conjunction with one or more others. These drugs may be killing stray cancer cells, or may be shrinking a tumor, or may simply be keeping a cancer in check. There are, after all, more than 100 types of cancer, and each will react differently. The manner of administration of chemotherapy differs. Some of the chemicals can be taken in pill or drink form; others are administered by needle; still others are given via an intravenous drip. Pills are most often taken at home by the patient. The other forms may need to be received in the doctor's office or in a hospital.

The problem with these powerful drugs is that in attacking cancer cells, they also do violence to healthy cells. Hence the problems with nausea, tiredness, etc., attendant on chemotherapy. For many, a serious side effect of chemotherapy is the loss of hair.

All these therapies and their side effects are prices we pay for cures, for improved health, to maintain the status quo, or, at the very least, to slow our decline. We should be communicating openly with our doctors to decide whether the price is worth the benefit.

*T*oday's
Recipe: Carpe Diem

I ended the first column in this series with the words *Carpe diem*. Many readers wrote to ask what it means. Forgive me. I thought the expression, although Latin, was better known.

The great Roman poet Quintus Horatius Flaccus, whom we know as Horace, and who is still a good read after two millennia, ends one of his odes: *Dum loquimur, fugerit invida aetas; carpe diem; quam minimum credula postero*. Or in English, "Even as we speak, time begrudgingly marches on. Enjoy today. Put as little faith as possible in tomorrow."

Literally, *Carpe diem* means "Seize the day", but my translation above conveys Horace's meaning better than the closer rendition. "Enjoy today" is really a powerful motto and a great idea. Another great scribe — I think it was I — wrote that today is the only day we have. Tomorrow never comes.

I saw a wonderful movie, *The Dead Poets Society*. Robin Williams, playing the inspired literature teacher in a prep school, frequently uses the expression *Carpe diem* to impress on his students the brevity of life and the need to use their time to the fullest and to maximize their lives.

Those of us who have terminal diseases have had the shortness of life impressed upon us. Our tomorrows are limited, so our todays become more important. Of course, we can do anything we want with them. We can hate today. We can be glum about it. We can sulk through it. We can be angry that we have another day with cancer or whatever. Do that if you want.

As for me, I'm going to have a dandy time today, and every day I'm given. I'm going to have a smile and howdeedo for every person I pass. And you know what? I'll bet every one of them says hello back, even the cute chicks who'll be wondering what this old lecher is all about. I'm going to enjoy every aspect of my job, because I can do it again, and still, and without the pain that plagued me months ago. I'm going to revel in the scenery, whether mountain or sandhill, river or gutter, castle or hovel, simply because it's there.

Yes, I'm going to enjoy today. I'm going to learn something new today. Maybe it'll be a few more words of Italian or of Spanish, or maybe a little more geography. Science has been at different times of my life a vocation and an avocation, but always a joy. Today I find myself learning a great deal about cancer and biology, particularly my own. My job, always a challenge, frequently and fortunately affords me the opportunity of gaining education in some trade or craft or business.

I'm going to do as much reading as possible, especially some of the good old stuff that I never read or have now half-forgotten. Several days ago I delved into some writings of the English Renaissance poet John Donne, whom I hadn't read since college, more than a few years ago. I was particularly taken by a strange poem entitled "The Flea" in which the poet celebrated the fact that both he and his beloved were bitten by the same flea, mixing their bloods in a kind of mystical marriage. A few days later a close friend reminded me that if I ever need blood, as I might, she is willing to donate. The love involved in the offer struck me, particularly in light of my rereading of Donne. I've always felt that nothing I've learned has been without value, but the applications are not always so quick in arriving.

Yes, I will enjoy today. I will admire the pretty girls who pass my corner. And I will listen to the sage advice of my elders, spurning much of it, but enjoying it anyway. I'll take great pleasure in keeping an eye on our greatest spectator sport, politics, realizing that it has changed very little since the days of Horace. I'll take every friend up on an offer to have lunch together, and I'll make a date right then. No more, "Let's get together someday."

Since I've had cancer, my main squeeze and I have forgotten the meaning of *mañana*. When one of us says, "Let's...," the other says "Yes" before the sentence is finished. This ailment has been a great learning experience.

The Latin poet spoke to us all when he advised us to enjoy today. It is a recipe for living, for all of us, those in good health and those of us who are not.

Carpe diem.

Patients
Must Learn Patience

*I*f my brief research into English composition is correct, the words *patients* and *patience* are both homonyms and homophones. That is, they sound alike but convey different meanings. Actually the two words come from a common Latin ancestor, meaning suffering, but *patience* has developed a much broader connotation in our language.

The past many months, however, have demonstrated to me that there is a close and essential connection between the two concepts.

But first, an aside about the terminology of sickness. I don't like most of it — the terminology, that is. (I'm not crazy about sickness either.) Yes, I have cancer, but I'm not sick. Indeed, I was sick during the summer, but now I'm quite well, working full-time and more, and enjoying life better than ever. And yes, I see my doctor every two or three weeks, but I don't think of myself as a patient. Patients are people in hospitals or confined to bed at home or in nursing care facilities. I also don't like the word suffering, as in suffering from cancer. I have cancer, but I'm not suffering. Nor am I a victim of cancer. Victims are what muggers and wars leave behind.

Now that I've made it virtually impossible to discuss any illness, let's try to proceed with, and about, patience.

Patience, acceptance, perseverance and forbearance are undoubtedly the chief virtues required, nay, demanded, of us who live with cancer. The term long-suffering was coined for us. The ailment does little for our sense of well-being, nor do the therapies that have become a part of the landscape for us. Chemotherapies, the medicines that keep us going, holding the cancer in check, also take a toll on our energies, drive, enthusiasm, ability to do what we want, our joy. Herein, of course, lies our greatest challenge.

Patience has never been an American virtue, particularly for us of the male persuasion. We are trained and conditioned to respect and admire accomplishment, or at least the appearance of accomplishment. We need to retool, as industry would have it, to rethink our concepts of what is really important in life. I've always liked the poem of Gerard Manley Hopkins, *In honour of St. Alphonsus Rodriguez, Lay-brother of the Society of Jesus*. Hopkins contrasts the glory of fighting men and the heroism of martyrs with "those years and years...of world without event that in Majorca Alfonso watched the door." The simplicity and holiness of the brother who spent 40 years tending the front door at the Jesuit house were of no less value than the work of his better known colleagues who made reputations for themselves as famous missionaries and scholars.

Most of us must now learn what else we can do. Just as at the beginnings of our working lives we took one path out of several we could have chosen, we again are faced with a choice of roads. Some are closed to us, including one or another on which we have already trod. No matter. We are all capable of many things.

It is very easy for us to feel sorry for ourselves and to focus on what we cannot do. When I see people jogging, I feel a pang of regret that I can never do that again. Of course, I then remind myself that it's been a quarter century since I did it last, and that I had no intention of ever trying it again. And I can feel bad that I can't ride a horse, but nothing in the past 15 years has induced me to get into a saddle. We have to remember that everything forbidden looks more attractive.

We mustn't overlook the positive aspects of our conditions. In my case, I'm prevented from lifting anything heavy. Often frustrating, to be sure. But think of what I can avoid. Christmas tree shopping? You're on your own this year, girls. Need help moving? I'll mind the truck. Not all bad at all.

Being the object of care, being in need is probably the hardest and most difficult aspect of our ailments. But there is a wonder and a beauty in allowing people to express their love to us. This has been the best part of the past many months. Knowing how much I'm loved has been worth the price.

*G*rateful
to Be Here

*M*y father had his first heart attack when he was still in his mid-40s. For the next 25 years he half-jokingly introduced the holidays each year with, "This will my last Christmas. Let's make it a good one." Finally, of course, he was right.

We who have terminal illnesses, and our loved ones, can approach days like Christmas with bittersweet feelings, wondering whether we will live to see another. As a health question, it's legitimate. As a way to celebrate a feast, it stinks. Every year can be an endless succession of birthdays, holidays, holydays, anniversaries, all remembered as potentially final feasts. Everyone, not just we who ail, can do this. So why not just decorate the front door with black crepe and leave it there?

Not I. I am a Christian and I will celebrate this most Christian of feasts with true Christian joy. Remember that it is the nature of a Christian to be joyous. Of course it might be my last Christmas — on this earth, that is. And if it is, then next Christmas will be so much the better. Christmas in heaven has to be celebrated better than we can do it here. For that I should be sad?

But for this year, at least, I'll be enjoying the feast here and be grateful. Grateful I'm here, grateful I can celebrate, grateful I have so many people who love and care about me, grateful I'm with them, grateful I can give and receive gifts and grateful for the health I have.

Yes, I am grateful for my health. My glass is half full. If it's also half empty, that's because I've already enjoyed half a glass, and for that I'm grateful too. And I will savor what's left, to the last delicious drop. Am I really dying? Sure I am. But we all are, from the day we're born. Just the other day a true philosopher commented to me that "Life's an illness, and there's only one cure." But we're living first. And as long as I continue to breathe, I'll use that breath to celebrate the life we share here on this earth, a good life, a happy life, made even better with the promise of an even better one to follow. So what's to be sad about?

Christmas is a time to be especially happy. For some folks holidays like this are a downer, but if we focus on the real, not the commercial, meaning of the feast, we can enjoy it. It is a time — a time, not a day — to celebrate God's love for us in sending the Messiah, Jesus' love for us in his birth, life, death and resurrection, his teachings and example. It is a time to celebrate the love we have, the blessings we enjoy. It is particularly a time to share love and blessings, for in giving, we will find ourselves richer.

Yes, this is a feast of giving, not of receiving. Love is not diminished in its sharing, but increased. Paradoxically, the more love we give, the more we possess. And the more we receive.

So I will celebrate this Christmas with laughter and love, with ample food and plentiful drink. And the next one will be better yet. Wherever it may be.

*T*his Doc Empowers Patients

*B*ernie Siegel is not your ordinary doctor. He urges patients to get themselves categorized as "uncooperative" in their medical files. It's probably not the recommended way of ingratiating yourself with your doctor, but making brownie points isn't where most of Bernie's clients are at.

Dr. Siegel is a New Haven surgeon who also teaches at Yale University. But it isn't for those things he's become known. Some 13 years ago he founded ECaP (Exceptional Cancer Patients) to make patients aware of their own potential to take charge of their illnesses. To Bernie (and he insists on being called Bernie, not Doctor), exceptional patients are those who accept cancer as a challenge, not as a defeat.

I recently took part in a two-day workshop with Bernie. The room of about 120 people was charged with power. About half were people with serious ailments, particularly cancer and multiple sclerosis, plus spouses, friends and caregivers. It was heartening to see the number of doctors, nurses and therapists there. Unlike the atmosphere in the usual cancer ward, doctor's office or clinic, there were few people that weekend who looked defeated.

Many had read Bernie's books, *Love, Medicine & Miracles* and *Peace, Love and Healing*. The workshop brought to life much of what is in the books. He imparts such power to patients that he has been accused of raising false hopes in seriously sick people. I encountered some people in the two days who did feel that they could permanently overcome any ailment. One man got quite angry with me for mentioning my own death. He felt I was admitting defeat.

Bernie, however, was not responsible. He started the workshop with the clear statement, "If you came not to die, get a refund. You're going to die anyway." And: "Don't eat vegetables to prevent death. You'll be mad when you get to heaven." Also, the final chapter of *Love, Medicine & Miracles* is titled *Love and Death*.

Bernie got into the business of helping patients help themselves when one of his patients told him, "I need to know how to live between office visits." He urges people to take charge of their own cases, finding doctors who will assist them, not the other way around. He is very critical of dictatorial doctors and doctors who do not listen to what their patients are telling them. Medical schools, he said, do not train doctors to listen. He recalled that Karl Jung made an important diagnosis by listening to a patient's story of a dream she had.

Being a medical doctor himself, Bernie is obviously not anti-doctor, but he insists that in addition to technical competence, a doctor must care for the patient as a person and leave room for the patient to make choices. Siegel keeps lists of such doctors and will share their names with people who ask.

Probably the most impressive thing about Bernie Siegel is his ordinariness. He does not come with a bag full of esoteric suggestions or remedies. Most of what he advocates can be described as just plain old common sense. He says himself that the best cures for everyday problems are found in "Mothers' Messages," such as "something good will come from this," or "if God closes one door, he opens another," or "nothing happens by chance."

(To be continued)

Message
Not Just for Ailing

*B*ernie Siegel sees his role as a doctor as half of a healing team. The other half is the patient. And they are both students, learning from each other.

This may not be the usual model of doctor-patient relationships, but Bernie Siegel doesn't fit the ordinary doctor mold either. Communication in both directions between doctor and patient is an essential part of the process, he insists. The doctor must be both technically proficient and a good listener. He is not dealing with a symptom, but a whole human person. If a patient cannot communicate with his physician, he should change doctors, Siegel says.

In *Love, Medicine & Miracles* Siegel describes the transformation that he underwent in the late 70s. He changed the way he practiced medicine, he wrote, becoming less a technician and more of a counsellor and teacher. He began to see his patients as part of the team.

He learned early on in this process that he, the doctor, needed healing as much as the patient. He took to hugging his patients to make them feel loved, but came to realize that it was often he who needed the hugs more than the patient. In the seminar, he commented that when things are not going too well between patient and doctor, maybe the doctor just needs a hug.

Bernie Siegel also accepts the anger of patients, because it means that the patient feels comfortable enough with him to show the anger. He then advises them to redirect the anger against the illness. He thinks it's wonderful when someone can get the anger out, be done with it, then live and love again. "It's great to dump the garbage," he said.

Doctors are often frustrated by their inability to cure patients, Bernie says. But curing and helping can be different skills, and doctors help patients when they empower them. And empowerment is what

Bernie Siegel does best, in his books and seminars and tapes. He helps people with serious illnesses help themselves, not only to get better, but to live life more fully, even with that illness.

Bernie's message is not just for the ailing, but for all of us. For reasons that I don't know, about two years ago, long before I knew that I had cancer, my favorite wife ordered several of Bernie's tapes from ECaP (Exceptional Cancer Patients). The tapes aid in visualization and hypnosis, two tools that can aid anyone in living more fully, so I was aware of some of the gospel Bernie preaches before I knew I was in such need of the message.

I've been very fortunate in my medical needs. For the last decade I've had a general practitioner who always listened to me, cared about me, and treated me as a whole person, not just as an ailment. He's not just a wonderful man, but an excellent doctor as well, and it was he who quickly diagnosed my cancer. He in turn referred me to an oncologist, whose office policy is to help the patient in the way the patient wants to be helped. With these two doctors and Bernie too, I'm in excellent hands.

ECaP is located at 2 Church Street South, New Haven, CT 06519. The two books mentioned above are available in local bookstores.

*N*on-traditional
Treatments

*T*ime was when I wouldn't have accepted any medical or health advice from anyone except an M.D. or an R.N. But I've grown too old and seen too much, and even learned from my experiences, to hang onto such conservative positions.

Many friends with serious back ailments that the medical profession couldn't help turned to chiropractors and found permanent relief. In recent years I've come to learn the potency of hypnosis to control mind and body and just a few months ago I opted to control my own high blood pressure with hypnosis rather than medication, with immediate and continuing success.

The ancient healing methods of the East are still considered novel here, and suspect by many, but acupuncture came to national attention back in the early 70s when President Nixon made his historic visit to China. Scotty Reston of the *New York Times*, probably the most respected columnist in the U.S., was covering the trip when he came down with a sudden attack of appendicitis that required emergency surgery. As the Chinese doctors did for everyone, they used acupuncture as anesthesia. Reston's story of the success of that method got many of us to thinking.

Not far from Boston is a place where anyone can learn about and experience myriad forms of healing, development, psychology, massage, meditation and spirituality. I'm tempted to say, as several others have, that some of what Interface offers is "far out", but I'm loath to be judgmental about things I don't understand. If someone is helped to cope with life and its vicissitudes, then whatever is helping them to cope is of value. Those of us with terminal illnesses are often in need of more than ordinary aids to deal with our ailments and their ramifications. Here, of course, we get into the issue of false hope, but that subject is very involved and difficult.

In the Health and Healing section of Interface's winter catalog are such offerings as: Dynamics of Food and Healing; Tongue Fu, using humor to combat stress; The Comic Within; Energy Healing; Vision Therapy; Illness as a Creative Response; The African Healing Dance; Therapeutic Touch; The Two Faces of Cancer; The Chronic Fatigue Syndrome; Myth and the Body, recovering the power to heal ourselves; With and Without Medicine, a map of the mindbody kingdom; Empowering the Caregiver; the Synergy of Belief and Biology, and more.

Members of the medical profession are among those offering courses at Interface. Deepak Chopra, also an M.D., frequently offers Interface courses on the old Indian natural medicine known as Ayurveda. I attended Bernie Siegel's workshop at Interface.

The catalog's section on Inner Development offers courses on handwriting analysis, healing for abuse survivors, keeping a personal journal, dream interpretation, understanding our prenatal lives, Milton Erickson, dealing with anger, decision making, loving ourselves, joy, self esteem, change in our lives, and forgiveness.

A variety of massage techniques are offered, as are courses in yoga and t'ai chi. There are several seminars on addiction and codependency. Women's studies occupies another section, and another is devoted to courses on maleness.

The Spiritual Inquiry section lists offerings in Insight Meditation, a Buddhist technique that is now frequently used in Christian retreats; the mysticism of Henry David Thoreau; the teachings of Krishnamurti; Kabbalah, the mystic tradition of Judaism; and North American Indian Shamanism.

R_{oot}
Hope in Reality

W_e have often discussed hope in this column. We who have terminal illnesses need hope — hope that our ailments can be cured or ameliorated or at least that we can maintain ourselves in comfort and dignity and without too much pain — and hope in a life that has a quality to it.

We've also discussed in this space the ways in which we can take charge of our lives and the methods of maintaining and fostering hope, like using good medical doctors, hospitals that provide qualified and caring nursing, support groups, a loving and nurturing environment, positive thinking, hypnosis, acupuncture and so on. The list is long.

Dr. Bernie Siegel and the late Norman Cousins have probably done more than anyone else to inspire people with serious sicknesses to fight and continue to live fruitful lives. But a disturbing corollary of this attitude is the feeling that positive attitudes can conquer all diseases. I'm not blaming either writer for the sins of their followers.

Hope must be rooted in reality. One reality is that each of us is going to die. A second reality for most of us with cancer is that the cancer will kill us. A hope that denies reality is, I believe, a false hope. Now Bernie Siegel, with whom I am in accord most of the time, calls the term "false hope" an oxymoron — a contradiction in terms. I disagree, respectfully though. Unfortunately, it exists.

As I've stated in recent columns, anything and anyone that supports and helps sick people to cope and deal with their ailments is good, unless in the end it is going to prove a disappointment and an illusion. This applies to every support from medical doctors to crystals.

A couple of months ago I spent considerable time and money locating a clinic in another country for a friend who is very sick with cancer. She had heard that this facility is performing "miracles" with some wonder drug. Shades of laetrile in Mexico a couple of decades ago! I located the clinic, and not unexpectedly was told by someone on the scene that it is nothing but a charlatan operation. You come, pay your money, and still die. There will always be such places — usually outside the U.S. — that seek to profit from the sufferings of others. And there will always be sufferers willing to try anything to stave off death.

I always knew I was going to die. Nonetheless, a new acceptance of this reality, and in a new time frame, was required when I learned last year that I have an incurable cancer. This acceptance has freed me in so many ways. I know, better than I ever did, who I am, where I'm at, and where I'm going. I can deal with myself, my doctors and nurses, the entire medical profession, my loved ones and whatever I choose to aid me physically, emotionally and spiritually, with no illusions or false expectations. Medical technology, prayer, meditation and hypnosis are all essential parts of my support system. So are love, work and my writing.

We each must find for ourselves those elements of reality that work for us. Locating our way is not easy, because proponents of one system look with a jaundiced eye on other methods. Medical doctors tend to have scant understanding or appreciation of anything that hasn't been tested by the Federal Drug Administration or approved by the American Medical Association. Everyone else has a litany of mistakes and failures of the medical profession.

We have a large smorgasbord from which to choose. If we choose well, and keep our feet planted on the ground, we'll stay happy.

Carpe diem — enjoy today.

Shopping for a Doctor

*T*he quality of doctors we have here in the Boston area is truly amazing. Absolutely nothing but the best. Everyone I know goes to a doctor who is "the very best in his field" or "almost a Nobel prize winner" or "usually you have to wait two years for an appointment with him but I was able to get in right away." Et cetera, et cetera, and et cetera.

One has to wonder where all the other doctors go. If my math is correct, half the doctors graduated in the bottom 50% of their class. Or, to put it another way, 50% of the doctors graduated in the lower half of their class. So where is the last half of each class, from each medical school? Have they all moved to Kansas?

Medicine, like any other profession, has its share of klutzes. Certainly the demand for medical school culls the field somewhat, giving the advantage to the brighter lads and lassies, but people who examine well but have trouble tying their shoes slip through. And get to be doctors. And specialists.

How do we find a good and competent doctor? There is no Consumer's Report to guide us. We have to rely on the recommendations of other doctors and of friends. And we have to use our own judgment and instinct. We must not be afraid to ask questions and make demands. It is, after all, my body, not the doctor's, that is under consideration here. If we don't feel comfortable with a doctor, there are a lot more M.D.s out there.

Those of us who have serious and terminal ailments are looking for more in a doctor than a quick fix for what is bothering us at the moment. Rather, we need someone to shepherd us through months or years of dealing with a condition that is not fixable and that will deteriorate with time and eventually be the agent of our deaths.

We want a doctor with excellent technical skills first. For some of us, that is sufficient. But most of us want at least a little coddling. We want someone who is understanding and compassionate and has some feeling for us at this difficult time in our lives. Unfortunately, it is not always easy to find a doctor who uses both head and heart to our advantage.

We have some of the finest hospitals and medical centers in the nation right here in the Boston area. But it is a mistake to presume that the doctors at those institutions are necessarily the best. Many of the most competent physicians prefer a smaller private or community practice, or want to work in a smaller hospital setting, or don't fancy the team concept of the large hospitals. We consumers should also look at the style of practice and pick what suits us.

When I learned that I had cancer I debated for several days over the style of oncology treatment I wanted. I opted for: 1) an extremely intelligent doctor; 2) in a small practice; 3) nearby; 4) who affiliates at a hospital not far from my home. In making this choice, I decided against: 1) a large practice; 2) a teaching hospital; 3) anything very far from home. I wanted one doctor in charge of my case, not several. I didn't want to be in a teaching setting because I knew I would lose patience being part of the education of young residents and medical students. I see my doctor often and didn't want to spend a lot of time traveling to and from his office.

Chances are I will be hospitalized with infection from time to time, and I want my family and close friends to be able to visit me easily. These are matters of personal taste, and we each must choose what makes us comfortable.

Also, as a former scientist, I want to know as much as possible about my condition and treatment. I want, and have, a doctor who answers my questions. This is not important to many people. Several of my friends with cancer want to know nothing. They simply do what their doctor tells them. I want to be part of the decision-making process.

Support Groups Important

I definitely didn't want to go. All my adult life I've hated meetings. And a support group was nothing but a meeting, I had decided. Besides, I had been dealing quite well with my cancer and was in no particular need of this type of assistance, I thought.

Fortunately the woman I live with works on different wavelengths from my own. She went ahead and made arrangements. She was going to go anyway and hoped that I'd accompany her. I spoke to the social worker at the hospital sponsoring the support group. She also wanted me to participate. Reluctantly I agreed to attend the first session, but would make no commitment for all six.

Half way through that first meeting I said to myself, "This is a good place to be."

There were five of us with five different cancers. There were also two spouses, a friend, a woman whose mother has cancer and the social worker. Throughout the half dozen sessions we each helped and were helped. The support group gave me a sense of not being the only one in the world with cancer.

Yes, I had discussed cancer and terminal disease with some others who have similar conditions, but I had never "rapped" about these topics in the same way, and with the twin goals of getting and giving. The group was what it set out to be — a support. We shared views, experiences, articles, and most importantly, love.

Yes, love. Though we were all strangers when we met, we formed close bonds very quickly. Those attachments outlasted the six weekly sessions and we've gotten together at a couple of our homes since. Some have met for lunch and we've had plenty of phone contact.

Over the past couple of weeks there's been a lot of phoning, because the sickest member of our group is about to die. We can all be glad that we gave her some support during her last six months of life. And that is what a support group is all about.

There are support groups for many, if not all, of the 100 or so different cancers that can affect us. There are support groups for women who have lost their hair because of chemotherapy. There are groups for people on the way to recovery and for families of cancer patients. Relatives of deceased cancer patients can find assistance. Some groups, like my own, were programmed only to last a set number of weeks; others are ongoing.

So how do you find a support group that suits your needs? Probably quite easily. First, ask your doctor, nurses, technicians and others involved in your treatment. Most of them will have recommendations. Then ask others who have cancer. Chances are they know of sources of help.

Also, the American Cancer Society (ACS) maintains offices all over the country. An assistant at an office near me says that they usually have a referral list of about 50 support groups that are operating at any one time. She said that most are either free or based on a sliding scale of payment, and that all but a few can be entered at any time. She added that the majority of them are located at hospitals and are easily accessible.

She said that the ACS office usually can also provide other assistance such as transportation for patients, emergency medicine and supplies, but that the funding for such services had expired for the year. However, the office is still supplying the referral service, as well as literature and educational programs.

We
Should Plan Ahead

*T*ending to the business of dying is not easy, but it's something that everyone should do at some point, both for ourselves and for our loved ones. We who have terminal diagnoses should do it without delay.

We should attend to three matters: a will, funeral arrangements, and the treatment we prefer when we are in our last stages.

We can leave our possessions to anyone we want, but the details MUST be in a legal will to ensure that our desires are carried out. It is not enough to tell Cousin Susie how we want the property distributed. Without that legal document, Susie will have no authority to do anything with our goods, and the provisions of state law will determine their distribution.

Anyone who makes out a will without benefit of an attorney is asking for trouble. Yes, it will cost, but the price is moderate and well worth the paying. You do not need the high priced services of the downtown law firms. Many small independent practitioners can handle the matter.

Making funeral arrangements for ourselves may not be the most pleasant task, but it is best not left until the day we die. Our survivors will have more than enough to do that day and do not need the added burden of a visit to the funeral director. Besides, most of us have particular desires regarding our funerals, so why not discuss their practicality and cost with the professional rather than with a relative who knows little more than we do about them.

Most of our local funeral directors (they don't like to be called undertakers any more — I refer to mine as my travel agent) are prepared to talk about advance arrangements and can set up pre-payment trusts.

Deciding on our care at the end of life can be very important. Absent contrary instructions from us, doctors and hospitals may feel a legal and moral obligation to prolong our lives far longer than we might want. For me, life must have a certain quality, without which I do not want to live. Once I have reached the stage where I'm beyond communicating, I want to die as quickly as possible.

There are two documents that should become operative at this stage. The first is a statement of our intentions as to what life-prolonging care we want or do not want, sometimes called a Living Will. Though never granted legal status by the Massachusetts legislature, case law — court decisions — has mandated that medical providers must follow the known desires of patients.

The second document, known as a Health Care Proxy in this state, and elsewhere as a Durable Power of Attorney, is really a backup for the Living Will and can supply for contingencies that may have been missed. This grants to another party the right to make decisions about our care when we are unable to do so. This type of document was given legal status in this Commonwealth. The legislation specified exactly how the proxy was to read. The details are simple, but an attorney should be consulted to ensure that it complies with the law. We obviously should also consult with the person named as our alter ego, to let him/her know just what we want. Remember, his/her decision will be final!

Keep in mind that neither document has any effect as long as we are of sound mind and able to communicate with our medical providers.

It is also not a bad idea to discuss these matters with our doctors and let them have a copy of the living will and the health care proxy. It takes some people by surprise that doctors frequently don't feel any more comfortable discussing death than anyone else. Remember that your doctor's job is, at least in part, to keep you alive. Your death can represent a personal failure for him/her.

Patients Are Caregivers

*L*ife is never simple, and that's good. It can be the complications that add spice and excitement. If everything were predictable we'd be bored. If we knew exactly what was going to be around the next corner, we wouldn't bother turning it. Or to put it another way, using the old canard, life is full of surprises.

Until my diagnosis I enjoyed more than half a century of quite good health. Like most other folks who walk this planet, I had an occasional bout with this, that, or t'other ailment, always brief, not terribly serious and quite fixable.

It was, therefore, a whole new ball game last year when I learned that I have cancer, and of the non-fixable kind. I had achieved the distinction of permanent patient, not something to which I had been aspiring. And it was hardly something for which I had been preparing. Or so I thought.

The word patient evokes images of someone lying abed, tubes entering or exiting several orifices and in places where orifices had not heretofore existed, nurses hovering, pills aplenty, doctors sagely nodding, et cetera. But many of us "patients" look just like everyone else. We walk, talk and take nourishment like the healthy. We may even be found in the local pub, or riding a bike, or taking a trip, or sailing in the harbor.

We who have terminal illnesses come in all sizes and shapes and colors and conditions, but we have two things in common. We need some special loving and understanding and attention. And we have all become caregivers.

Yes, caregivers. Because now everyone close to us, everyone who loves us, is in need. They all need exactly what we need: love, understanding and attention. They, after all, are about to lose someone they care for. They will be experiencing a sense of loss that we will not know.

This caregiving role took me by surprise. I had always assumed that it was the folks with the ailment who needed the care. But, of course, I never walked in these shoes before. I suddenly saw this group of saddened humanity around me, all close friends, all in need of consoling. I found that I had a special role to play in offering them comfort. Only I can assure them that I'm fine, that I will be fine, and so will they.

In most cases it is up to us to initiate the discussion, because very few people can bring up the subject of another's death. (I still have trouble with that.) We must do it. And then we can help each other. We can learn about each others' fears and sorrows and most importantly, plans. I say plans, because the fact that we're talking indicates that we're still living, and no matter what our condition, we should try to make each day as full and happy as possible. What do we, patients and those we care for, want to do to maximize each day we have together? It is only by talking frankly that we can plan together whatever days we have left.

We can, of course, bewail that we have only X number of days remaining, or we can rejoice that we have so many days, and try to make them the best yet. Or the best they can be. That way, we'll leave our loved ones with more than money or homes or cars or trust funds. We'll bequeath them wonderful memories.

And one of the best memories they'll have of us will be of those last days or months or years when they were taking care of us. Or so they'll think. They may never know that we were really taking care of them.

Friends Are the Best Medicine

*A*ll too often we think of medicine as what comes in bottles. But medicines were around long before bottles. We who have serious and terminal ailments get exposed to more medicines — and here I use the term medicine in its widest sense — than we ever knew existed. There are tens of thousands of pills and capsules, liquids to be swallowed, injected, dripped or applied. There are the mysterious and invisible x-rays and electron rays. Acupuncture needles help many. Hypnosis, prayer, meditation, diets, baths alleviate many sicknesses.

Yet there is a medicine more powerful than any of the above, less expensive than all, always available and with infallible curative powers. I've been taking heavy doses of it recently and I've never felt better. What is it? I speak of friendship.

Recently an old, but not close, friend, whom I see infrequently, called just to see how I was feeling. That touched me very much. During that week two of my closest friends called from their homes in New Mexico and California to chat. Since I see them so seldom, our telephone conversations are precious.

I'm penning these words at 35,000 feet en route back to Boston from Jamaica, once my home, where I've just spent a week enjoying the company of many old friends. It was one of the most wonderful weeks of my life. And that has nothing to do with the popular image of Jamaica. In fact, my bathing suit was never out of my suitcase. Except for the rides to and from the airport, I never saw a beach. What I was there for was to bask, not in the fabled Caribbean sun, but in the love of friends. And that I did.

Yes, I'm aware that, given my condition, this might have been my last visit to Jamaica and that it may have been my farewell to some of these friends. But whether this was the ultimate, or penultimate, visit does not really matter. What counts is that we were together, that we laughed, that we enjoyed and that we loved. How many more times we do it is not important.

Nor is it vital that good friends be in physical proximity. We live in each others' hearts. My own peripatetic existence, and that of many I love, has left me with friends scattered around the world. Often years, and sometimes decades, pass without us meeting. But then conversations take up where they left off. That's what friendship is all about.

Is my cancer improved because of this luxuriating in friends, as I've been doing? Probably not. But I am. I'm happier, more relaxed, more energetic, and just better all around because I know I'm loved. Can I ask any more?

I always knew that something would kill me. For the past nine months I've been pretty sure that this cancer would be the agent. But our focus cannot be on our deaths. It has to be on our lives. And our friends are the most wonderful part of our lives. They do for us so much more than medicines. There is no treasure greater than a friend.

Imperfection Is a Virtue

*T*hat I am a flawed person has long been an important part of my personal philosophy. In my two teaching episodes, one in secondary school and one in university, I tried to impart to my students that we are all very imperfect beings.

I think an appreciation of our built-in shortcomings is essential in our quest to understand ourselves. It particularly explains why we fail to achieve all we want and set out to accomplish. It helps to absolve our many mistakes and errors. Rather than be discouraged when we cannot become the person we want to be, we can take solace in the fact that our inabilities are indwelling and God-given.

Of course, we must not use this as an excuse for not trying, for it is only in seeking to reach beyond our capabilities that we test our limits — that we continue to grow.

A long, long time ago I accepted the fact that I would never make an 18-foot pole vault or a six-foot high jump or a four-minute mile. In more recent times I reconciled to not knowing a dozen languages, never becoming editor of one of our major metropolitan dailies, or of being a noted scientist. The list of my inabilities is long.

So ten months ago it did not come as a major shock that I had more imperfections than I had known. When my doctor told me I had an incurable cancer this was just added to the long list. It did not constitute a first flaw in a perfect person. Friends tell me I took the news and live with it well, and I believe that's true. In thinking into my acceptance, which has been easy, I see several reasons, but I think that my old philosophy of imperfection is at the core.

People who think they're perfect have obvious problems, as do those who cannot accept their failures. Yet of all animal existence, it takes man longest to be capable of freedom from the nest and we are more dependent on our fellows than any other beast or bird. The colds, flus, aches and pains, the minor and major ailments that from time to time bring most of us to a doctor are all reminders of our frailty and mortality.

So my fatal disease is really just the capstone and confirmation of what has preceded and what I had always known. It is not the end, but rather a new challenge, a time once again to test my capabilities. Within this new framework of living with disease that will eventually mean my demise and which even now imposes certain limits, I still have many goals, and some of them are related to the ailment. Some I will achieve and some I will not. But the fun will remain in the trying.

And my death will not be a failure. It will be something very different.

Enjoy *Today*

I was somewhat saddened the other day to hear one of our veteran talk show hosts ask listeners to consider what they would do if they got the word they had a limited number of days to live. How would they make each day count as much as possible? he asked.

Newsflash, dear reader. You have a limited number of days to live. That's a fact. Now start making every day count. Make each one the best. Push yourself to the max. Be your happiest. Live life to the fullest.

Why should you wait until your doctor tells you that you have an incurable cancer, or that your heart is giving out, or that your diabetes is out of control? Are you going to wait till then to start living? Do you really need a brain transplant?

Regular readers of this column are aware, I hope, that I'm writing primarily for others who, like me, have serious and terminal illnesses. But I'm writing about living, not dying, so my message is for everyone who's still living. As St. Augustine said, we all suffer from that serious illness called life, and there's only one cure for it. Each day from the moment of birth we're a day closer to death. So let's get the most out of life!

As I've mentioned before, the Latin poet Horace has long been one of my favorite reads. I've been particularly fond of the 11th ode of Book One, in which he says we mustn't try to learn when we're going to die, but that we must enjoy today, never trusting in tomorrow. That's the origin of his famous words, *Carpe diem*, which is literally translated "Seize the Day", but which is better rendered as "Enjoy Today."

I've been most fortunate in having had a very happy life. A concatenation of people, places, times and events have given me 54 halcyon years. I would have had to reject much of what was presented to have had anything but enjoyable days. Part of the philosophy that I developed was a focus on the today, the only day we ever have. Tomorrow never comes, and yesterday is history.

This philosophy stands me well today, now that I have a better fix on how limited my time on this earth is. While each day has long been precious to me, there is an added value to each one now. And that value involves all who are closest to me.

When I got the news, almost a year ago now, that I have a terminal cancer, the one thing that bothered me most was the sadness my death would bring to my family and friends. There first seemed nothing I could do about it. But reflection taught me otherwise. I could assuage their tears, I could lighten their heavy hearts by leaving them happy memories. The memory of how I enjoyed my days with them, the thoughts of our laughing and our loving, will outlast the mourning.

So my enjoyment of today is not just for me, but for a host of others. And the fun is in being with them, today in body, later in spirit.

Carpe diem! Enjoy today.

Emotional
Help May Be Needed

*M*any of us need more than medical assistance when we learn that the affliction that has our attention is the one that will, in all likelihood, end our lives. Depression, anxiety, fear and consideration of suicide can require psychological, psychiatric, spiritual, emotional or some other kind of mental adjustment.

I had a brief discussion the other day about the head problems of the terminally ill with Dr. Ned Cassem, Chief of Psychiatry at Massachusetts General Hospital. My conversation was brief only because I had agreed — and I kept my bargain — that I would take only 15 minutes of his time. Given my druthers, we would have talked for hours.

Ned made a decision years ago to spend as much time as possible with patients with the worst illnesses because "I learn so much from them." He is disappointed that so few in his profession have shown interest in the spiritual and psychological aspects of suffering and what death means to people who "stare it in the face," as he put it.

Ned Cassem feels that the first obligation of the psychiatrist treating a terminal patient is to learn what the patient wants. For many, he said, death is not the problem. "What comes between now and then is a major problem." The pain, the discomfort and particularly the need to depend on others are what scare people.

Many think of themselves as worthless burdens on their families. They see their lives as having lost meaning. Some then see suicide as an option. Ned finds that the medical doctors of many such people have not paid attention to what the patients are saying. Often they've been requesting advice that has not been forthcoming.

Ned said that much can be done to restore the self image of such patients and to enhance their sense of worth. And a great deal can be done to allay their fears of the future.

He praised the work of the Sloan-Kettering Cancer Institute in New York, where "the alleviation of pain has been raised to an art." He thinks that one of the basic duties of the physician is to relieve suffering, "maybe not back to the baseline," but to make the patient comfortable.

Ned said he is willing to administer morphine in sufficient doses to relieve pain, even if this renders the patient unconscious. This can also lead to death. Patients are comfortable with the promise of such treatment, he said.

Dr. Cassem spoke at some length of the need of the terminally ill to rely on others. "The ability to depend on others is a higher form of maturity," he said. People see it as one of the real threats to the integrity of life.

Ned said he keeps learning the answers to such problems from his patients. He said he has seen quadriplegics who were destroyed by their incapacity. "Others did such a job dealing with pain it has blown me away." He said he's found many role models in his dealing with the very sick.

After 24 years in the business, Ned Cassem said he doesn't have a lot of answers, but he keeps trying to learn — from patients. And he continues to help patients develop their own answers.

My head's been pretty straight in the year since I learned I have cancer. But if I need help I know where I'll go — if Ned could fit me into his incredibly busy schedule. In addition to his full-time job as Chief of Psychiatry, Ned Cassem is also a Jesuit priest.

A Year
of Learning

My writing was never intended to be about me, nor has it been, though readers have learned quite a bit about my thinking. However, I've decided to make a report about my own health, because this week I celebrate the first anniversary of the day my doctor told me I have an incurable and a terminal cancer. A year already! Time does pass when you're having fun!

I say that only partially facetiously, because these past 12 months have been at the same time the most difficult, the most challenging, the most adventurous and the most wonderful of my life. Those four adjectives probably belong together and form a symbiotic whole.

The diagnosis did not floor me. Several things had been going wrong in my body over six months, so I, having some slight and general knowledge of science and medicine, had already considered cancer as one of the possibilities. Then, too, the pain in my back had reached such an intensity that I would have gladly accepted any diagnosis that would lead to alleviation. (In retrospect, I only thought the pain was bad then. It was to increase tenfold over the next couple of months before it would start to diminish.)

My diagnosis was of multiple myeloma, a bone marrow cancer, which untreated, attacks the bones; in my case the spinal column and ribs particularly. The bone marrow is the blood factory, so the blood my marrow produces is and always will be defective. Most critical here is the white blood count, because elements of the white blood cells fight infection. About 60% of people with this cancer die of infection.

I spent a very long weekend deciding whom to choose for an oncologist. I debated long and hard between the teaching hospitals, Massachusetts General Hospital and Dana-Farber particularly, and a small practice. Distance from my home was a factor. I picked a doctor who was recommended for his brilliance and his caring, and that's exactly what I've found him to be. The staff in his office, which includes a lab, are so thoughtful and nice that I look forward to my twice-monthly visits.

Seven weeks of daily radiation had a large role in knocking down my pain, though it was six months before I was able to terminate pain medication entirely. I took so much morphine and Percocet last year that I had visions of agents from the Drug Enforcement Administration knocking on my door.

All I'm left with now is minor achiness in my lower spine. The cancer has left me with a damaged spine; I have osteoporosis, so I dare not lift anything heavy lest I create another compression fracture, undoubtedly the cause of much of my pain last year. (I'm almost two inches shorter than I was a year and a half ago.)

Friends and acquaintances who see me for the first time in a year always expect to see someone looking weak and debilitated, and indeed I did look that way last year. I had to use a cane for many months. But I look perfectly healthy now, and I feel generally healthy most of the time.

I've resumed gardening and bike riding, two pleasures that I had thought were history for me. Would it be safer to avoid these activities? Sure, but I'll have a long time when I can't do them. I refuse to wrap myself in a protective sheath. Life is still to be lived, and as fully as possible.

The most wonderful part of this experience has been the love and care that my family and friends have shown me. I never had any reason to doubt their affection, but it's been manifested so often and in so many ways that at times I feel smothered in love. Not a bad way to go! I've made so many new friends, often people like me who are coping with cancer. I've drawn much inspiration and courage from them.

The cancer is still at work in me. Monthly chemotherapy keeps its activity at a low level, and I may enjoy a few years of this moderately good health. The average life expectancy with this multiple myeloma is 3–4 years. My doctor expects I'll be on the long side of that. The chemo exacts a small price, mainly fatigue and a further depressed white blood count, exposing me even more to infection, but the benefits are worth it.

No matter. I don't fear death. Nor do I any longer fear the approach to death, because pain and distress can be managed. I will enjoy today, and each of the todays I'm granted. I will continue to enjoy the daily learning about medicine and the lab work in my own body, marvelling at what science makes possible. And I will continue to enjoy my daily work, particularly now that I have no worry about the future of the business. Fear and worry and fretting are gone from my life.

Carpe diem! Enjoy today!

Considering Chemotherapy

*C*hemotherapy has a bad reputation. And not undeservedly. I know of no one with cancer who looks forward to the next chemo treatment. I certainly don't. There are side effects that are less than pleasant.

But it's worth it. For me anyway. And that's what it's all about. Is the price worth the gain? That's what each of us with cancer has to ask ourselves.

If the cancer is curable, or has a pretty good chance of being eliminated, there isn't much to debate. Of course you go with it. But there are other considerations for those of us with cancers of the incurable type. A couple of my friends, recently diagnosed with cancer, decided against chemo because they've seen others who've suffered with it. I'm not sure that their decisions were properly made.

Chemotherapy is the introduction of cancer killing chemicals into our bodies. Unfortunately most or all of these medicines attack more than the cancers, causing what we call the side effects. Many of us suffer declines in white blood cell counts, opening us to infections. Most of us get tired. Nausea is common during or after chemotherapy. I get irritable, then very tired for several days. That's all. The chemo keeps my cancer at a fairly low level. My health is generally good. My lifestyle is normal. I probably have a few extra years. I pay a small price of a few days of discomfort for all these benefits. For me there's no choice. Of course I'll continue on chemo.

For others the price is steeper and the benefits may not be as great. This is something that each patient should discuss in great detail with the doctor. What will life be without chemo? What will the chemo do — for good and bad? The answers may not be too simple and clear cut. Each of us reacts differently to cancer and to chemo. For most of us there are a variety of medicines that may work, each offering different progress and problems. There are about 50 medicines used regularly to treat the hundred or so cancers, plus scores of others that are in experimental use. There are also myriad medications to counter the side effects of chemotherapy. A good oncologist will be willing to answer all a patient's questions about the possible treatments. If he isn't, find another doctor, no problem here in the Boston area.

The administration of chemo may be anything from an intravenous drip during a hospital stay to taking pills at home. Many go to a doctor's office for an hour or two of an IV drip. Chemo is given to some people only a few times. Others of us take it on a regular basis.

If chemo is an option, talk to your doctor, talk to your relatives and loved ones and make a choice based on the length and quality of life the treatment offers. If you want to try it, remember that you can always change your mind.

Death
Rate Is Constant

Death rates for some diseases are down in this section of Boston, according to some figures I saw during a recent meeting at Carney Hospital. A committee on which I serve was presented with a lengthy list of death rates from a variety of ailments and the up and down movements of those rates from year to year. Interesting, and informative about a lot of the lifestyles and health problems in our neighborhood.

But at one point I said to myself, "Whoa! The real death rate is 100 percent. Everyone in the study area, and everywhere else, is going to die."

Sometimes health professionals give the impression that death is about to be conquered. We get statistics on the decline of cancer rates, or on death from heart attacks, and we think that real progress has been made. Logic dictates that if the death rate from cancer goes down, death from something else has to rise. And that's because the death rate has to remain at 100 percent, and no scientific advances are going to change that.

Of course, in the past many years the average age of death has been pushed back dramatically. The "miracle drugs," as we called them back in the 40's — penicillin and its cousins — had a lot to do with this. Health care in general and nutrition plus better understanding of our bodies with resultant improved lifestyles have been major factors in increased longevity. When I was a kid, not very long ago, few people reached 80. Now octogenarians are legion. An example. Back when I joined the Jesuits in the mid 50's, only three or four New England Jesuits a year celebrated a golden jubilee. This year's catalogue of the New England province lists two priests in the order for 70 years, 10 celebrating 60 years, and 14 marking a half century. Every one of the golden jubilarians is still working full time.

All of this, of course, has given rise to a new field of medicine — gerontology. Which is another way of saying that we now have
a whole array of new diseases. They're probably not new, but not many
people lived long enough to manifest them. Alzheimers disease is just
one of them.

The rise in the number of nursing homes in the past couple
of decades leads one to wonder if medical research and care is doing its
job too well. Many of us are living beyond our usefulness. And there is
every indication that the need for geriatric beds will continue to grow.

There are serious economic ramifications to all this. The care
of the elderly, many of whom are receiving public assistance, is becoming a major financial problem. The social security system was designed
in a time when many of its contributors didn't live long enough to collect anything, and the majority of those who did collect did so for only a
few years.

Some of us who are told we have a fatal disease and only a
limited time to live feel cheated, as though we're being singled out. No,
death comes to us all, and to each at our own time. No one really dies
early. There are many advantages, both to us and to society, if we die
"with our boots on."

*L*ife
Is Sacred

*I*t's no secret that one of the best selling do-it-yourself books around now is a manual on how to commit suicide. I'm not really happy about that.

I've never heard truly compelling philosophical or theological arguments against suicide, so I'm not about to condemn the practice. But I'm not in favor of it either. Philosophy and theology don't have all the answers, after all.

I can understand someone facing a messy, painful and difficult death considering suicide as an option. A friend of mine has AIDS and cancer. The depressed immune system due to the virus gets in the way of cancer treatment, and life becomes more trying every day. He's contemplating suicide and I'm saying nothing to dissuade him. However, the cancer at work in my own body gives promise of a death less attractive than what I might choose out of a catalogue, but suicide is not in the cards for me.

As readers are aware, I hold life and living in high regard — sacred, really. When I grow tomatoes and corn and daisies and roses I participate in creation. There is no way I could take a healthy flower or fruit and step on it. I'm a carnivore, but I would never kill an animal just for sport.

Human life is much more sacred than that of plants or animals. All societies have held such life as special and have demanded stiff penalties of those who wantonly murder.

There is much that is beautiful and wondrous in the conception and birth of a human. Few events evoke as much joy as the birth of a baby. Death should be no less wonderful and awesome, even though it causes a natural loneliness and sadness on the part of those left behind.

The origins of life have been the focus of much dissension in recent years. Abortion is, of course, the big battle ground. But the most ardent pro-abortionists of my ken don't LIKE abortion, but accept it as a necessity. Various methods of artificial insemination and surrogate parenting have also been the subject of ethical debate, but I see no great movement to deposit sperm and eggs in a central lab for implantation into the most eugenic wombs. The natural methods will continue to appeal.

There is something sad about people who are unable to cope with the challenges of this world, whether it is a teenager perplexed by the prospect of adulthood or someone refusing to accept the death he is dealt. Suicide is failure. Suicide is a very selfish act, and leaves family and friends with an added burden of grief. And it is at center a life destroying action.

As mentioned earlier, someone who has a fatal disease has many options other than suicide. Medical science can provide fair freedom from pain and discomfort. The act of dying may not be a day at the beach, but I can't see running from this any more than from any other uncomfortable moment in life. Or should we recommend suicide whenever the going gets rough?

The problem with the new suicide manual is that it will encourage more people, and make it easier for them, to fail, to quit.

Dying is no less a challenge than living. It is, indeed, part of the living process. Facing death, and accepting it, is one of life's supreme challenges.

Joy
Is Medicine

*T*he daily papers recently carried an interesting piece about a British medical study that indicated people under stress are more likely to come down with the common cold.

Since the study of about 600 subjects focused only on the virus that causes the all-too-common cold, scientists cannot extrapolate to other viruses or to bacteria. But we can make an educated guess that further studies will demonstrate that stressed people are subject also to other germs.

So what's the big deal, you might say. Why, in a column dealing with living with terminal illness, are we getting excited about colds? Simply because the new study supports and reinforces what I've contended many times — that one's mental attitude has a profound effect on physical health. This is true for everyone, but has deeper implications for those of us with serious illnesses.

Year by year the evidence of psychosomatic health builds. Not only can the mind cause ailments, but it can prevent and cure illness as well. Of course, beyond that, happy and well adjusted people are able to deal with sickness better than grouchy and sad people. Hippocrates, the father of medicine, wrote about the healing power of joy. Many of his followers, long before today's scientific methods were devised, also recognized that happiness is curative. Today we're just starting to learn about endorphins, a morphine-like chemical that is secreted in the brain during laughter and exercise and which induces feelings of well-being and even of creativity.

Maybe the message here is that we who have terminal ailments should simply work at making ourselves happy, if indeed that should be called work, and let the doctors take care of the rest. I took some heat from some of my nearest and dearest for going out on foot and on bicycle during Hurricane Bob. But I thought: why am I keeping myself alive with medicines if not to walk in hurricanes? There has to be more to this cancer than just surviving till the next round of chemotherapy. We who are terminal can afford a devil-may-care attitude much more than others. And why not? What have we to lose? In a lot of ways we who are on limited time have been freed from many of the fears and worries that plague our "healthy" brothers and sisters. That, of course, raises the interesting question of what is health in the first place.

Just last week my doctor asked, somewhat incredulously, if I were not coming down with infections, as I am "supposed to", given my condition. I answered with a simple "No." Maybe my answer, with explanation, should have been, "No, I walk in hurricanes instead."

Yes, given the opportunity I'll walk in another hurricane, and I'll continue to sail and walk in the woods and do detective work and ogle the girls — all potentially dangerous activities — because they make me happy. And probably healthy too.

Carpe diem. Enjoy today.

A Fighter's Story

Some two decades and more ago my favorite columnist was Max Lerner. He was carried by one of the Boston papers and by hundreds of others across the country. Writing about current affairs from the perspective of historian, political sociologist, literateur and philosopher, Lerner was a true renaissance man, bringing the wisdom of millennia as well as his own inspired insight to his observations on the passing scene. He was at the same time a college professor, teaching at Brandeis, Sarah Lawrence and Notre Dame, among others. And along the way he penned some 14 books.

Lerner never slowed down. A dozen years ago, at the age of 78, he was still engaged in a full schedule of teaching and writing. Suddenly his life changed. First he discovered he had cancer. Then, while he was still fighting that ailment, a second and different cancer appeared. And a few years later he had a heart attack. A year ago Lerner wrote still another book, *Wrestling With the Angel: A Memoir of My Triumph Over Illness*.

The book is named after the Genesis story of Jacob spending a night wrestling with an angel, after which he declared, "I have seen God face to face, and my life is saved". Lerner, a religious man, also came face to face with God in his illness. He accepted death, while fighting to live.

This is the marvelous story of a nonagenarian who is still a student, but now, instead of politics and civilization, he learns the mysteries of his own body and of his own ability to conquer the ailments that besiege that body. Lerner fathomed that the most important healer was the "doctor within" — the marvelous ability to heal himself. The support and love of his wife and five children were major factors in the healing process.

Lerner, who is the father of Adam, a doctor (now at Dana-Farber Cancer Institute here in Boston) and of another son, Michael, who is engaged in "alternate" therapies in California, took from both. In his workshops and seminars he had dealt with holistic medicine. In this book he insisted that the imagination and will can fuel the sense of the possible to cure the body.

At the same time, Lerner obtained the best medical assistance he knew. After careful and prolonged consultation with his doctors he opted for chemotherapy, and against radiation. For the second cancer, he chose an experimental medicine to avoid problematic surgery.

But most importantly, he remained in charge of his own treatment. While respectful of the superior medical knowledge of his doctors, he always made the final decisions. The very fact of being in charge played a large role in Lerner's success over the cancers and heart ailment.

Lerner's is a wonderful book, both for the well and the ill. It is of special value for those who care for the sick. Lerner's reflections on the feelings and needs and goals of a patient bear reflection. He also shares many insights on death, having been deepy affected by the death of a brother when he was nine, and by the death of his own daughter at the age of 29. These two events strongly colored his thinking as he faced his own mortality.

This is the story of a fighter, and of a winner. The word helpless is not in Lerner's vocabulary. I hope that he's at work right now on a sequel. Ad multos et plurimos annos, Max.

[Author's note: Max Lerner died a year after the above article was written.]

As
Natural as
the Sunrise

During the past couple of weeks several events have conspired to force on me thoughts of death, my own and others. To some, this might seem like very negative thinking, but in the 15 months since I've known I had a terminal cancer, my death has come to be as natural as tomorrow's sunrise, and I fear it no more than that. To others, of course, my death will seem an end, but to me it will be a passage.

My doctor said that after the next cycle of chemotherapy, probably in early November, we will suspend treatment for the time being. In my case, this indicates that the cancer has stabilized, not gone into remission. No gain will accrue from further treatment at this time. We'll watch it monthly and when it gets more active, resume the chemo. This step was a reminder that I have come so far down a road, and that there is only a certain distance left.

I attended the funerals of two friends. First, there was the service for Steve J., who had AIDS and cancer. He was 47, and growing up gay when he did was very difficult.

Steve's relations with his parents were always very poor, and he had trouble relating to others as well. About a year ago I asked him what he wanted from the rest of his life, and he replied, "I just want to be happy." Happiness, unfortunately, was a quality that eluded Steve his entire life. It is only in death that he has found it.

A couple of days later I went to the wake and funeral of Mary Murphy, who used to live on Crockett Avenue here in the Dorchester neighborhood of Boston, but has been south of the city in Hanover for about 15 years. Mary and Gene were a very happy couple, and they raised three beautiful daughters who have stayed close to each other both emotionally and physically, living within just a few miles of each other. The daughters' six children relate as siblings, rather than as cousins. Though we all missed Mary we celebrated the rich life she had, together with the wonderful memories she left. And now she has greater happiness.

Then I met a 26-year-old woman who, in the course of our first conversation, mentioned that she has a terminal cancer. She relates to her ailment as I do to mine, and has similar views on the quality of life. She is totally open about her cancer, and tries to live every day to the fullest. She's staying in school and preparing to be a hospital chaplain. I found in her a true soulmate. Two days after we met a friend handed her a magazine article he thought would interest her. It did, but for reasons he hadn't anticipated. It was something I had written!

Another reminder of the wonderful reality of death came in a letter from an old and dear friend, Paul Horgan, a missionary priest out in Ponape, in the South Pacific. "I'd like to see you again," he wrote, "but I'm not due back in the States until maybe the summer of 1993. However, if not then, then a bit later." In the scheme of eternity, it will be only a bit later.

At Steve's funeral service, a woman read a passage from an unidentified source. It compared death to a sailing ship passing from us to the horizon. The ship is in no way diminished because it grows smaller in our eyes. It is only we who suffer loss from its absence. But just as we say, "There it goes," on the other side of the water are those who say, "Here it comes."

Carpe diem. Enjoy today.

Healing in Advance

*P*rophylactic medicine is one of the most important aspects of the healing art. The word prophylactic, associated by most laypeople with condoms, derives from the Greek, meaning to guard against something in advance. Thus, vaccinations and inoculations are prophylactic. Dentists call the annual or semi-annual cleaning and check-up prophylaxis.

A couple of years before I moved to Jamaica, the government had begun an anti-malaria campaign which included the occasional inspection of every toilet on the island. The result is that there hasn't been a home-grown case of malaria in Jamaica in over 30 years now. The great success story in prophylactic medicine is smallpox, which, about ten or a dozen years ago, was completely eradicated from the face of the earth.

Now this is a bit of a roundabout way to introduce my topic. Over the past 15 months since my doctor told me I have a terminal cancer, I've reflected a lot on my reaction to the news. It was not what the experts tell us it was "supposed" to be. I didn't feel anger, fear, bitterness, frustration and all the other emotions that are said to be normal reactions to such news. According to Doctor Elisabeth Kubler-Ross and others who've written on the subject, a certain amount of psychological healing usually precedes acceptance of the fatal diagnosis.

Why did I not need that healing? Why did I accept the news with immediate peace and tranquility and even happiness? How could I do the mental transfer from a state of lifelong robust health to that of a fatal illness without some serious adjustment? These questions have dogged me for over a year, and I certainly don't have all the answers, but I think I know some of them.

Probably a healing process is required, but I think I received my healing prophylactically — in advance. The intellectual and spiritual training I received, together with the very healthy emotional atmosphere in which I've fortunately lived my entire life, all contributed to my acceptance of a fatal diagnosis.

The nurturing, the loving, the strong self-image that are needed by the sick have been my constant companions. Inner peace and a sense of humor are also important elements of my life. A supportive network of family and close friends all these years gave me the strength to see myself as no different from the person I had been prior to the knowledge of my cancer.

Of note, and of importance to all of us, both the ailing and the well, is that none of what I see as my prophylactic healing came through licensed or professional caregivers, but through the ordinary contacts through life with family and friends. This makes us all caregivers of others, an important and challenging role. We often don't know how much good we're doing when we reach out and touch someone with a bit of love. Just ask me.

We
Are All Healers

*T*here's a lot of hurt going around.

Last week I attended a single night of the parish mission at St. Gregory's church at Lower Mills here in Dorchester. The theme of the evening was healing. At the end of the service everyone had the opportunity to have one of the three Franciscan Friars who were conducting the mission pray over them. My guess is that about 80% of the 600 people in church that night got in line.

I spoke to several people. All the ailments weren't physical. A lot of people are carrying psychological burdens and scars. We who have only physical sickness have the easier time of it.

One of the friars made the distinction between cures and healing. Cures are what the doctors do across the street from the church at Carney Hospital. Healing goes much deeper. And you can have one without the other. Curing is often easy. Healing is more difficult, and much more important. It's great if you can have both.

We all should be in the healing business. Unfortunately many of us are responsible for the hurts of others. Most psychological ailments are imposed by others, particularly adults doing a number on children. Kids are so delicate, impressionable and easily hurt. Healing from childhood ailments can be a lifetime's task.

In our busy, crowded, hard-working society it's all too easy to focus on ourselves and forget about others. Selfishness, unfortunately, is one of the more serious, and debilitating ailments of life in these parts. But it behooves us to think of others, first with a view to not harming others, and secondly to help salve the wounds of others, to help them carry their burdens.

Each of us, regardless of our own troubles, can reach out with a kind word, a smile, a hug or a kiss or an "I love you." Often we don't know who of our friends is in need of such balm, so we'll never know the good we do reaching out like this.

But we will have some idea of how much good we do for ourselves, because we're going to feel better about ourselves and because this treatment comes back to us. As we reach out to heal others we find we're healing ourselves. And everyone's better off.

If we can all start thinking this way, those of us with terminal and incurable ailments may not be cured, but we'll experience healing. And then the lack of a cure won't really matter.

Carpe diem. Enjoy today.

Giving
Thanks

The holidays are coming! Thanksgiving and Christmas, the two biggest family days of the year, can be bittersweet for us who are terminal and for our loved ones. We're all thankful that we're still here and we have to wonder if this will be the last one.

As I pointed out earlier some time ago, such thinking is silly. Every son and daughter of a mother on this planet has the same right as we to wonder if this is their last holiday season too. No such morbid and melancholy pondering for this son! Holidays are to be enjoyed, and enjoy them I will.

I have so much to be thankful for this year, probably more than ever before. This is my second holiday with the cancer, but this year I'm grateful that the pain that was still with me last year has receded to nothing but a dull ache.

I'm thankful for my wife, Barbara, and daughter, Laura. Long ago they extracted a promise from me that I would not write about them. So I'll write — of myself — that no man was ever more blessed in the women with whom he shares his home. I'm a very happy person, and they are the two biggest reasons.

My two brothers and four sisters are another cause for gratitude. They've always been there for me, always supported me, but their love and help has never been more felt than during the last year and a half. Five of the six of them live within a half mile of my house, and we continue to have a lot of fun together. Their several kids are now a very important and wonderful part of the mix.

I'm thankful for my two doctors. My primary doctor for many years, who is also a friend, diagnosed my uncommon cancer very quickly, thus affording early treatment for the increasing pain. He recommended an oncologist who's brilliant, caring, professional, even nice, and very importantly, he's allowed me to remain in control. Also, his associates, the nurses, technicians and receptionists at his office make a visit there both joyous and a reason for confidence.

I'm grateful for all the readers of this column who've spoken to me about my thoughts and told me how some idea of mine supported them or helped a friend. I thank those who've invited me to speak, giving me a chance to press the flesh with an audience. I thank Eddie Forry, the publisher and owner of this paper, for giving me the chance to communicate my thoughts in each issue, as well as for being a trusted and great friend. And I thank Sue Asci, the editor, for her professionalism, her broad and deep journalistic talents, her brilliance and wisdom and caring attitude, and especially for her friendship and love. And I thank her in advance for not excising that last sentence.

I'm thankful for each sunrise and sunset, for each day's light and darkness, for the sun and the rain and even the snow. I enjoy the passing waves of friends, and the bustle and joy of Adams Corner, the shopping area and heart of my neighborhood, and all Dorchester. As I've said many times, I'm not afraid of death, but I'm not rushing toward it either. I'm enjoying every day I'm here.

So on Thanksgiving, join me in thanking God for all we have. *Carpe diem*. Enjoy the day.

*T*oday
Is the Only Day

*O*ne of my first reactions to the news that my days on this earth were to be counted in low numbers was that this cancer had robbed me of my dreams. No longer could I envision what my very significant other and I would be doing in years to come. I was not to enjoy my daughter's success in a career nor probably hug my grandchildren. The completion of a novel I had started became problematical, and images of future novels dissipated. I then knew that my business would never develop in any other direction. Dreams of what can be have always inspired and fueled my actions, and I felt a little cheated.

Yes, the cancer has stolen many tomorrows from me, but it made me a wonderful gift of today. I always had a decent appreciation of living in the moment, but I never savored each day as I do now. Nor did I ever dream that there could be such satisfaction in the living totally in the present.

I often recall the wine drinking advice of a little French friend of mine. He scorned those who knock back a glass of good wine. "Just take a drop or two," Antoine said, "and let the taste roll around in your mouth." I've tried it with wine, and it works. Now I'm trying it with life, and it works there too.

Though I've earned gold medals in procrastination, the word *mañana* — tomorrow — has disappeared from my vocabulary. When the idea of calling up a friend comes to mind, my fingers stroke the buttons of the phone. No more are such thoughts consigned to future agenda. When a buddy and I agree to meet for lunch, we set a date. No more, "I'll call you soon."

I find myself stopping to have a word with people more often, instead of the passing "Hi Howaya". Even for just a moment or two we ask after each other and inquire about the other's family. We bless or curse the latest weather, which here in New England always provides a topic of conversation, then go on our ways, each a little richer. I try not to turn down any invitation to a gathering of friends, because I enjoy watching and taking part in the interplay of words, ideas, emotions and love.

As much as I relish the company of others, I cherish a certain amount of solitude too. I'm happy in my own company and with my own thoughts. I guess I'm happy with myself. I learned to accept myself many years ago, with all the warts and blemishes and imperfections that I can never cure. (I'm not sure I want to remedy them all.) I suppose that acceptance of the me who is, not just the me who might be, prepared me for this moment of todays without a lot of tomorrows.

While I still don't know if my novel will ever be finished, I've never derived as much satisfaction out of my writing as I do now. Writing these lines forces me to reflect on my life, and I find I like both the life and the reflection. I particularly like the feedback I get from those who've been touched by a word or thought I've expressed. All scribes derive satisfaction from being read, and more in being appreciated.

The tomorrows of the dreams of yesteryear have turned into yesterdays. Many of the dreams were fulfilled, while others were not, but even better than the dreams were the surprises. But they all were fulfilled on a today.

Carpe diem. Enjoy today.

Fellow Travellers

Some very special Christmas greetings: *

To Jackie. You've suffered so much these past few years, but always with a smile and with so much patience. You ask for nothing and give so much to those around you.

To Margaret. You told me of your recent mastectomy as though describing what you cooked for Thanksgiving dinner. Your courage defies words. I've never told you what your wonderful smile means to me.

To Bill. We discovered our cancers at the same time, but you've travelled a much rougher road than I. We've been through some other wars together, but none like this. You inspire me with your fearlessness and your buoyance.

To Charlie and Ed. We all found ourselves with the same cancer at the same time. Thanks for sharing all your thoughts and feelings and experiences with me. We've each chosen a different treatment. May they all work.

To Frannie and Pat. You've had my cancer for years, and you've given me hope, inspiration and your friendship.

To Bob. You took your relapse with such grace, and your suffer treatment the same way. We've found a kinship in our ailments and you've given me a model to follow.

To Sandy. Your determination to beat this thing is awesome. If medical science matches you, the game is won. Seeing you fighting with, and for, Phil and the kids is wonderful.

To Uta. You display such vitality and composure. Getting this melanoma the second time after you thought it was history must have been devastating, but you are so positive.

To John. You seldom mention your cancer. But just seeing you gives me a boost.

To Frank. You accepted your cancer as casually as the daily mail and you continued to work as though the disease were no more than a cold.

And to Marilyn. We walked together for a while. I know I was able to do a bit for you before you left us, but your fight, your humor and your friendship helped me more than you ever knew.

And to Steve. Cancer and AIDS dealt you a double sucker punch, and I know you found it a pretty tough end to a life that was never easy. Finally you have the happiness that always eluded you.

And to Joe. You were the first man I knew who could talk about his own death, and you brought such wonderful humor and courage to your last days, and to all of us who knew you.

And to John. You tried so hard not to let it beat you, knowing all the time that the battle with the disease would be a losing one, but your battle with life was a winner. The Alcoholics Anonymous principles that guided your recovery from alcoholism gave you so much help in the fight with cancer. The humor, and ability to laugh at yourself, that kept you sane in the earlier battle also guided you to the end. I miss you, John.

You all are proof that we don't walk this earth, or its twisting paths, alone. Each of you has helped me along, many before, all since I knew I had a terminal cancer. I can give you little except my thanks and my love.

*Written at Christmas 1991.

*W*ake
Up and See

*H*alf a lifetime ago, when I was a chemistry teacher, I started each new class with an instructive exercise. I gave each student a candle, with directions to write as many descriptive items as possible — look, feel, smell, taste were all to come into play. They were then to light the candle and continue to describe it, and finally extinguish it and add any further new descriptions.

I had assembled a list of more than a hundred items that catalogued the three states of the candle, but many students were hard pressed to detail a dozen. Few offered more than 25. The exercise, of course, was to train the students to observe, but it left me with a lasting lesson in how most of us sleepwalk through life.

We are surrounded by so much that is beautiful, interesting, fascinating, consoling, and even by some ugly and disgusting things too. Most of us never see or observe what is around us, as a starter, and secondly don't reflect on the qualities. That's what I call sleepwalking.

The first three months of the year are a dangerous time for many who find them cold and dreary and even depressing. The sun and warmth and growing things that buoy us at other seasons are missing. We are devoid of saving holidays during these months. Those of us who are further burdened by serious and terminal illnesses are apt to compare our time of life with the season.

I issue this clarion call to my fellow patients and to everyone else — AWAKE! WAKE UP! Make yourself alert to all the wonderful people and scenery and events and birds and clouds and rain and snow and love and care and laughter that surround us all. The beauty is there. Often only the beholder is lacking. Come spring and summer other sights and sounds will please us, but see what this season has to offer. See what TODAY brings.

Too much of what most of us read, and I am certainly guilty here, and most of what is presented on the boob tube, is geared to blank and dull our minds, rather than to educate us and turn us on to reality. We who must deal with the breakdown of our bodies are in particular need of reality therapy. Escaping to la-la land only makes it harder to face what is sometimes harsh.

But facing all the reality around us, the beauty and the wonder and the great, gives us a perspective in which to view our ailments. It is very easy for us to become self-centered and to begin to believe that our cancer or our failing hearts or minds are the totality of our existence. They are not.

So, class, your exercise for today is to take every single thing you see and hear and smell and taste and feel and ferret out the beauty of it. And then enjoy it.

Carpe diem. Enjoy today.

The Spirituality of Illness

*S*ome reflections on the spirituality of illness.

It's no secret that we can grow and become better people through adversity. The working out of problems, the need to accept situations that we consider less than ideal, and the realization of our own frailties and imperfections all can contribute to making us wiser. Each crisis in our lives should conclude with us knowing and liking ourselves better.

There are no problems like health problems. We can walk away from other difficulties, but our health is rather firmly attached to us. There is an essential difference between problems that are external to us and those that cut to the very essence of our being. High on that latter list are terminal ailments that promise a permanent change in our status as well as less than ideal living conditions in the meantime.

We can react to the news of a terminal or otherwise serious illness with confusion, anger and hurt, but those are probably the same emotions of animals below us on the evolutionary scale. Or we can, using all the human facilities at our disposal, work towards an understanding of who and what we are and where sickness fits into the grand scheme of our lives.

As a start, the birth, life and death of every person, as well as of all organic matter, is part of the constant renewing of the earth, a sign of the freshness that is deep down in everything.

Then, too, sickness, particularly the terminal variety, forces us, or should force us, to look into ourselves and evaluate what's important in our lives. If our priorities have been misplaced, we can correct them for whatever days remain. No point in bemoaning the mistakes of the past. Just live every day to the fullest.

Those of us who believe in a God and an afterlife (there can't possibly be one without the other) are also challenged to make ourselves fit for the journey to come. For many of us that might mean squaring things with others here with whom we have quarrels.

This is also a time for serious reflection on our relationships with our families and friends, what they mean to us and what we mean to them. It is a time for us all to express love without shame or embarrassment or reservation. It is a time to celebrate life. We must help our loved ones to accept our sickness and eventual passing, and give them an example to one day emulate when their own time comes. And we must leave them with wonderful memories of ourselves.

The joy of living need not be dampened by thoughts of death, but death should be seen only as a part of, and an affirmation of, life. And for those of us who know we're going to a better place, there is no end of life, but only an improvement.

These days bring new challenges and new excitement. I earlier referred to my new adventure. It has been and remains so. And it grows more exciting and fulfilling all the time.

Carpe diem. Enjoy today.

Details
of Patients' Rights

*O*ne of the things I like best about Christmas time is meeting so many new people at parties. This Christmas past I had the pleasure of making the acquaintance of Terry T., a young woman in whom intelligence, beauty and niceness seem to be competing for supremacy.

After we had discussed and solved many of the world's most pressing problems, we got to talking about patients and their treatment by doctors, nurses and particularly hospitals. Terry has been a health professional for several years and had much to say on the issue, about which she felt strongly.

Most of us let ourselves get pushed around somewhat, by bank tellers, supermarket clerks, shoppers in department stores, fellow riders on the rapid transit, the IRS, the clergy and our paperboys or girls, to name but a few, but there is no situation in which we feel so powerless as when we are in need of medical care. When we're sick we are also apt to suffer from fear and apprehension, which emotions can be exacerbated by a hospital setting, where we're told what to do, when to do it and how we are to do it. Or worse, we're told very little.

In the context of this conversation, Terri mentioned a professor of hers at the Boston University School of Public Health, George Annas, author of *The Rights of Patients*. She spoke of her great respect both for Annas and for his book. She obtained a copy for me.

Annas, an attorney, teaches health law both at the School of Public Health and at the Boston University School of Medicine. His book is one in the "rights" series of handbooks sponsored by the American Civil Liberties Union. Although I'm often critical of the crusades of the ACLU, I have nothing but praise for Annas' book. The author writes not from any antagonistic viewpoint, but in a vein that presupposes that the health system will work better if all know their rights and duties.

Some of the chapters deal with: the patient rights movement, the organization and functioning of hospitals and the rules that govern them, admission and discharge, informed consent, surgery and emergency care, pregnancy and birth, research and human experimentation, medical records, privacy and confidentiality, care of the dying, autopsy and medical malpractice.

The major message of this work is that patients remain in total charge of themselves and their medical care as long as they are of sound mind, and that they have the right to refuse any and all treatments. Annas helps patients understand the myriad consent forms they are asked to sign in a hospital, as well as the obligation the medical suppliers have to inform patients of the implications of all procedures.

The book also contains suggested forms for a living will and a durable power of attorney, and directions on the use of medical and law libraries.

Annas in an excellent writer, quite comfortable with his material, which he handles fairly informally and sometimes humorously. For instance, in dealing with the rights of patients to see their medical records (yes, you have the right) he cautions that deciphering physicians' handwriting may be a major hurdle.

Despite the fact that the book is written for laypeople in language we can all understand, it is full of such scholarly apparatus as footnotes and a list of other reference materials for those who want to pursue particular issues.

The book was published in 1989 and is a complete remake of a previous work put out in 1975. The publisher is the Southern Illinois University Press, PO Box 3697, Carbondale, IL 62902. It costs about $9.

*P*roductivity
at the End

*B*ernie Siegel, the New Haven surgeon who, through his writings* and lectures, has done so much to empower cancer patients, insists that a great many important truths are revealed in what he calls "mothers messages".

Examples are such as: "Nothing happens without a reason"; or, "God's looking out for you"; or, "There's no waste in God's economy"; and, "We all have a purpose in life".

Some might argue that these are just pious platitudes, but a counter argument can be made that such dicta remain in common usage only if they continue to manifest truth and reality.

Recent events have forced me to do some serious mulling about God's plan for the universe, Her plan for me, and my plans for me. The concepts of Fate and Divine Providence continue to pervade my thinking.

A year and a half after my diagnosis of cancer, I decided to leave the private detective business, which had been my major profession for a decade and a half. I wasn't sure what I was going to spend my time doing, but I knew I wanted to work more at helping people. Only three people knew of my decision.

Four days later I got a call from an old friend, Father Bill Raftery, the rector of Campion Center in Weston, just 20 miles from Boston. Campion is a Jesuit retreat house, residence, retirement home and health center. Bill read me a letter that had just been issued by the local provincial superior, announcing his decision to turn the Campion Renewal Center from a retreat house that focussed its attention chiefly on religious and clergy to one that caters mainly to the laity. Bill was offering me the post of assistant director, to work with him in running the place, recruiting retreatants and giving an occasional retreat. Bill had no idea that I had made a decision to change professions!

He was aware that over the previous year and more I had directed a couple of retreats. Is there more than coincidence with my growing interest in spirituality, my decision to change professions and the creation of this job?

Then there were my years of writing news and features about a variety of people, subjects and businesses, most eminently forgettable. Couple that with my background as a Jesuit, a teacher and a scientist. Add the newspaper for which I'd been writing a column for more than three years. Then enter my cancer and the decision to write a second column about life with a terminal illness. I find I'm doing the best writing of my career and having the most impact. Did all this just happen by chance?

It's very easy for us who have serious and fatal diseases to feel we're has-beens, castoffs, without purpose, nothing but a bother and a drain to other, younger, healthier people. Oh yes, I know the feeling. I remember thinking of myself as "damaged goods" when I first learned of my cancer. Little did I realize that I was entering on a period that was to become the finest, happiest and most productive of my life.

Many might find it odd of me to describe in such glowing terms what is also the last period of my life, but it seems that all I have done and learned is coming to best fruition now. I feel that everything else was aimed at this time, to converge into a symbiotic whole. It is as though all else was prelude for this moment.

Each of us, healthy and ailing, must continue to take stock of our lives and our progress through life, attempting to maximize each moment, making ourselves and our loved ones as happy as possible. We each will do it in different ways. I'm doing it for myself. I can't tell anyone else how to do it, but I remain convinced that we can all find happiness in any set of circumstances. Start now.

Carpe diem. Enjoy today.

* *Love, Medicine & Miracles* and *Peace, Love and Healing*

Searching
for Quality

I've been asked many times if I have tried macrobiotic diets, faith healing and other less than mainstream attempts to cure my incurable cancer. The answer is no. Many who have cancer, and even more who haven't, think that every possible or probable attempt should be made to effect a cure. I respectfully disagree. Following are some of my reasons.

There are many ways to deal with cancer. There is, of course, radiation, the use of which is very closely controlled, regulated and licensed. Then there's chemotherapy: about 50 medicines are in regular use and probably several hundred others in experimental use. Surgery is also an option for many cancers.

Mainstream medicine has also come to accept the positive thinking process as espoused by Dr. Herbert Benson at Deaconess Hospital in Boston, the author of *The Relaxation Response*, and Dr. Bernie Siegel of New Haven, author of *Love, Medicine & Miracles*. The two pioneers utilize their techniques only in conjunction with standard treatments. I'm a fan of both doctors.

At Dana-Farber, as well as at several other hospitals, experimental techniques are being employed to treat my cancer, none of them at this moment notoriously successful. Is there a chance that one or another would result in long term remission? Sure there's a chance, but the odds are also high that I'd suffer some long term disability from the treatments, including very long term death. Each person with cancer has to weigh the cost against the probable benefits and make a decision. I've made mine. I'm staying with the conservative and standard treatment that will probably give me a few years of comfortable, profitable and enjoyable life.

Beyond this are the chemical and other treatments that are available, usually outside the U.S. borders. Remember the laetrile "cure" in Mexico years ago. You can still find charlatans who will take the money of desperate people. I know there are people who claim that macrobiotic diets do wonderful things for cancer patients, but the American Medical Association has been unable to document the success of such treatment. Of course, I've had readers write me about the conspiracy of the AMA to keep many cancer remedies from the public because doctors would be out of work if a cure were found for cancer! That type of thinking boggles my mind.

Many are surprised that I haven't tried faith healing. I'm not disparaging it or trying to dissuade others from approaching it, but it just does not fit my style of spirituality. If God wants to cure me, He knows where to find me. Besides, we're in regular contact. And remember, He is the same God who let me get cancer in the first place.

People who remain convinced that there has to be a cure for their cancer, whether from medicine, prayer or will power, seem to forget that they have to die of something. An individual ailment might be cured, but death from something will still get us all in the end.

I feel that I have better things to do with whatever time I have left than continually search for the elusive cure. And I have better use for that time than simply trying to extend it. I'm having too much fun living every day.

Carpe diem. Enjoy today.

Limitations

*S*ome time ago I talked with a musician who was getting hard of hearing, and a man with a heart problem that had forced him to curtail both his activity and his once legendary appetite.

So what's the big deal, you say. There are still lots of other things they can do. To which I add a fervent Amen.

This reminds me of a friend, John Chapman. A cancer forced the loss of Chappie's lower right arm. Rather than bemoan the fact, he was thankful that he had had his hand for some 73 years. The last time I saw him, Chappie was telling me of all the things he was learning to do one-handed, and he asked me to hand him a cigarette. The operation had not gotten all the cancer, and he died shortly afterwards.

It is very easy for any of us with disabilities to bemoan what we can no longer do. But if we look realistically at ourselves, we have to recognize that we are all born with numerous disabilities. There are lots of things that others can do that we can't, due to accidents of birth, upbringing or temperament.

Life is much more productive and happy if we focus on what we can do, on what is available to us and then maximize our potential.

I say all this particularly to others, who, like me and the two mentioned above, have lost powers already enjoyed. A loss is probably harder than never having had a faculty. No matter, like Chappie, it's then time to be thankful for what we had as long as we had it, and learn new ways of operating. New challenges should be taken as opportunities for growth, not as impossible demands made on incompetents.

We can view ourselves as crippled if we want, but that's just a way of focusing our attention on our disabilities. And if we think of ourselves as crippled, then that's just what we will be. I find it more challenging and more fun to pay attention to what I can do. It's much more satisfying.

When my doctor told me that I have an incurable cancer, I had no idea that the challenges of dealing with the cancer and with the restrictions that it puts on me, would open so many doors and bring so much richness to my life. Had such notions been posed to me at the time I would have said that I was looking for no challenges. Thank God for surprises. They're part of the spice of this life.

Carpe diem. Enjoy today.

Community
of Care

Going public with my cancer was not an easy decision. I knew at the time I'd be giving up considerable privacy. I've learned that the need to write forces me to remember my ailment at times, like now, when its relative dormancy permits me to forget it for longer or shorter periods. So it's cost me something.

But I've gotten much more in return than I've surrendered or given. I've met some of the most wonderful, most loving, most exciting people on the face of this earth — people who have cancer or other life threatening diseases and others who have fought and conquered those ailments. I feel as though I've been admitted into a very special club.

One day at a social function, I introduced myself to an attractive young lady in her mid-30s. She knew me immediately as the author of my columns, and said she had used them in a support group at Massachusetts General Hospital. That, of course, told me something about her. We swapped notes for a quarter hour on our treatments and our hopes and our plans, and ended with a loving hug. Never have I found friendship and intimacy so easy and meaningful and helpful as it is in this "club".

A few minutes later I was in a similar conversation with a friend of some six months, a 24-year-old woman who's been told she has only a couple of years to live. Armed with a firm belief that she knows more about herself than her doctors do, she continues to prepare for a career, though her studies are sometimes interrupted by the roller coaster ride of chemotherapy. She loves reminding me that if the cancer wins, at least she won't have to repay her student loans! She always gives me courage.

A few days earlier I'd run into a friend of many years who revealed to me for the first time that she beat cancer more than a decade ago. She is one of so many people I've known for a long time but who have concealed their present or past bouts with the ailment. I've been admitted to a kinship.

Some while ago my wife and I were in a support group for six weeks, but we've continued as a social group that gets together for food and drink from time to time and to continue to support each other. Two of the original group have died, but some of us were able to help them in their last days.

It's hard to describe the empathy, the caring, the solicitude and the love that I've found in this new community of mine. I meet folks of enormous courage and strength. Many of us, in facing our physical ailments, discovered wellsprings of fortitude we never knew we possessed. And so many are willing to share these gifts with others.

We've also had to face one of the great truths of this life, that it ends, and had to deal with all that means. Most of us had to reorder our priorities, and it's not all bad to realize what's important and what's not, and to live in accordance with that knowledge. I now live in a community of people who know how vital it is to enjoy today, and how to do it. It's a lesson that everyone should learn at an early age.

I'm glad I went public with my cancer because I have so many good friends I never would have known at all, or known so well. I also urge anyone who's hiding cancer to share the secret with others. You'll find that you have a large support group among your present friends, many of whom, you'll find, share your ailment. Just like members of Alcoholics Anonymous, we're everywhere, and ready to help.

Carpe diem. Enjoy today.

Letter to a Friend

*D*ear_____

It's almost two years now since we learned that I have a terminal cancer. It's certainly been an interesting time. And a very good time, in many ways.

The problem is, it's been a much better time for me than for you. As you're keenly aware, I've been very happy, content, accepting, satisfied and fulfilled. Even in the days of the worst pain or the most aggravating chemotherapy, I did fine. Today, with my condition stabilized and chemotherapy suspended for the moment, I even forget my cancer for long periods. There's too much else that's fun and challenging in my life.

You, however, are not doing as well as I. When you see me, you see a guy who, in your mind, is about to buy the farm, kick the bucket, say goodbye. When you look at Ed Madden, you see a fatal cancer. When you hear my voice, you wonder how I am. You're angry about my condition. You're sad that I'm going to leave you one of these days. You get depressed about it. You feel powerless.

There is, of course, a difference between us. When I die, I'm going to a place of peace and happiness where suffering and sadness are against the law. If I'm wrong in my calculations and there is no God and no heaven, then I'll become part of nothing, where there's still no pain. You, however, will be here without me. And there will be a certain grief in that, at least for a while.

The problem here is that you're starting to grieve much too early. I am, after all, still with you. *Scribo, ergo sum.* I write, therefore I am, to misquote one philosopher. Or to paraphrase another, celebrate while the friend is with you; do your fasting and sorrowing when he's gone. Otherwise you'll later have two sources of grief: that I'm gone, and that you didn't enjoy me in my last years.

So, my friend, adopt that dictum of the poet Horace that I've taken as part of my own code: enjoy today and put scant trust in tomorrow.

Enjoy my company as much as I'm enjoying yours — for today. I take great pleasure in every moment that we spend together, in our conversations, in our understanding, in our shared joys and sorrows. I enjoy you because you are here in my life, today. I enjoy giving you of myself, and sharing in your life and your love. I'm very grateful for your presence in my life. It has always meant much, but so much more in these days. Enjoy the fact that you are such a support for me.

So, rather than burying me before I'm dead, let's hoist a few jars together this summer, or even a 'cuppa' java, share some tasty food, walk in the sunshine and just be together whenever we can. I have some new challenges in my life, quite apart from my ailment, that I'll tell you about — and sometimes even bore you with them. But we'll both enjoy the chat. I'm meeting so many new people now that I need to schmooze about them with you. I'm living, I'm loving my life, I'm so happy and I want you to share in this happiness of mine.

And yes, one day I will leave you. But I promise to leave you with a lot of happy memories.

I love you. *Carpe diem*. Enjoy today.

Ed

*T*he *Business of Living and Dying*

I was asked to address a group of business executives recently about my present place in life, my writing of this book. I accepted the invitation readily but then wondered what I would say to this audience. "You too can make money from terminal ailments."? Or maybe, "We're a growing segment of the population. Be sure you get your market share." Somehow this didn't seem like the right message.

I was joking with a friend in Toronto about these thoughts. He answered quite directly, telling me to give the business folks the same message I regularly try to communicate in my writing. "Businessmen more than anyone need to examine what they're doing and where they're going. Their lives can be wasted in their business," he said.

I realized then that the message I've been trying to impart to others who are terminally ill is probably the best thought that I could leave with the business men and women. They must learn to enjoy today.

We Americans are the envy of the world when it comes to business and industrial accomplishment, to getting things done, and to living well. But in discussions with Italian friends on a visit to their country, I found them laughing at our work habits. Many of us Americans have only two weeks vacation, and very few have four. But in Italy, most workers start with four, and within a few years have seven, eight, nine or ten weeks a year to do what they want. Many in Rome asked me what it is we're working for.

I'm not sure I have the answer to that question. What are we working for? Probably 90% of us would answer the same way: "I'm working for my family." But all too many of us are spending so much time providing money for our husbands, wives and children that we deprive them of what they really want most: us. In many cases we work so hard that we deprive ourselves of ourselves. We fail to do what we really want. We have to deal with many necessities, but economic necessity is only one of them. Other needs are more personal and more important: emotional, family, spiritual. What is the real legacy we want to leave our heirs? Most of us who run businesses are very good at prioritizing at work. Do we do so well at home?

In what may be a first for me, I'm actually taking my own advice. For the past 16 years I've been a private detective. I work for, and by, myself. Virtually all my clients are lawyers, and most of their clients are businesses. I spend a good deal of my time solving problems of these companies, many of them of their own making. I've enjoyed my work all these years, finding it challenging and exciting. It's been a constant learning process, because of the constant exposure to new businesses and industries and trades. It's been perfect for a perpetual student like me.

But since I've known I have a fatal cancer, I've changed and so have my interests. My writings have taken on a life of their own, and this has brought about work with the ill and their caregivers. As a result, the detective work has taken second place in my work life.

When I told my wife and daughter and a couple of close friends that I was going to close my agency, I wasn't quite sure what I was going to do, but knew it would be in the area of human and personal service, something that would bring me more in touch with people and their needs. Four days after I made this announcement I got a phone call from Father Bill Raftery, the rector of Campion Center in Weston. He told me that the retreat house there was converting from a facility geared to priests and religious to one catering to the needs of the laity. Would I be interested, he asked, in joining him in that work?

I did not take long to answer yes.

So at a time I had not expected to still be alive, I'm starting on a new career, a career which I hope will help others face themselves and their God and help to put their lives in perspective.

Carpe diem. Enjoy today. I am.

Life's a Mess

*B*ob McMillan is the best preacher I know, and I'm not alone in that opinion. He always has something to say and he says it well. Bob is a priest and the rector at the Jesuit Urban Center in the South End of Boston.

One Sunday Bob was talking about the mess God made, and how he, Bob, would have done it better. Why, he asked, did God create a world beset with black flies and other bugs in the summer months when we all want to be outdoors. Bob, if he were the creator, would have allotted the bugs the month of February, when we stay indoors as much as possible! Makes sense to me. Next time there's an election for God, I know who's getting my vote.

Bob's words, as usual, left an impression on me. His ideas about the mess that this world is jibe with my oft-expressed philosophy that we humans are very imperfect creatures. Acceptance of these concepts makes life, and its vicissitudes, a lot easier.

As a start, couldn't God have thought of an easier way to get us born? Talk about mess! And childhood — so much work for parents. The teen years are so anguishing for both kids and parents. Why didn't God just produce us as perfectly formed and perfect adults?

I don't know the answer to that. I just know that he made us pretty flawed. And a world full of people prone to mistakes does make for quite a mess.

If we accept that we are damaged goods from the start, and that this world is somewhat less than it might have been if Bob McMillan had manufactured it, then we won't be surprised or taken back quite so much when serious illness strikes us. I've said before that I think my long standing recognition of my own flawed nature stood me in good stead when I learned that I have a terminal cancer. The only news was that I was a little more damaged than I had realized.

I think that people who seek and expect perfection in themselves or their environment are bound to be disappointed throughout life. They live in expectation of what cannot be. Serious illness can be devastating for them.

I'm not suggesting that we should welcome news of fatal or serious diseases with either joy or indifference. Such announcements are bound to be upsetting. But sickness is not an aberration or distortion of the natural order of things. It is natural.

When Bob McMillan was preaching on Sunday, I couldn't help but think of the humerous sign I've seen in so many homes: God bless this mess.

Carpe diem. Enjoy today.

T_{wo}
of the Best Years

I threw a party the other night. As parties go, it was a great one. About 25 of us, each others' closest friends and most of us related to each other, gathered at my house where, for more than seven hours, we ate and drank and laughed and loved. There wasn't much to update with each other because most of us see all the others every week anyway.

This party was very much a celebration of love and closeness and sharing and helping and just of being with each other. It was the anniversary of my diagnosis with an incurable cancer. A couple of the less reverent in our group referred to our gathering as a "cancer party" and "the carcinogenic party". Whatever you call it, it was fun.

There was a lot to celebrate. I had good reason to believe I wouldn't be here now and certainly not enjoying my current relatively good health. I know that the place in which I'm going to end up is supposed to be a lot better than this place, but this place is the only place I know, so I'm quite happy to stay here as long as I'm functioning normally.

We celebrated our closeness and our love. We've always been close, but my cancer has pointed up for all of us the brevity and fragility of life, and we "seize the day" a little better because of our heightened awareness of the blessing of having, and being, friends.

I was celebrating the completion, and continuation, of the best years of my life. That may sound somewhat ridiculous to some readers, but those who have followed my writings know the appreciation of life to which this ailment has brought me. And those who know me well know how I've been smothered in love by so many these two years. That, of course, doesn't mean that I wouldn't rid myself of the cancer if that were possible.

We could, of course, all spend our time cursing my cancer and bemoaning that my days on this earth are coming to an end. And we could go on from there to regret every bad thing that happened to every one of us, and every day, week, month and year that weren't up to our expectations. And we could continue to grouse about all the evil and suffering and problems we see around us every day.

But, you know what? It's a lot more fun to party. It's infinitely more satisfying to count our blessings. I remember an old philosophy professor of mine at Spring Hill College down in Mobile, Alabama, Father Joe Bogue, commenting one day that the singer Eddie Fisher spent some time every evening counting his blessings. Then Joe added, "Of course, he goes to bed every night with Elizabeth Taylor!"

Each of us has, and have had, problems and pain in our lives. But there's a lot of good that happens to us too. Without being polyannaish, it's healthier and certainly much more satisfying to concentrate on the good. That's what I do, and I'll continue doing it. And then I'll throw another party to celebrate.

Carpe diem. Enjoy today.

I Can't
Beat This

"You'll beat this thing; I know you will." "You'll be just fine; I'm certain of it." "You'll still be here 20 years from now."

I hear such remarks often, from friends who are expressing their hopes for me, rather than the realities of my situation. I will not beat "this thing", the terminal cancer that invaded my body, and I will not be here 20 years from now, or 10 either. I will however be fine, but not in the same sense my friends mean it. I'll be fine, but elsewhere.

I've never been bothered by such comments, as I understand the good will that's engendering them. But some of my friends who also have terminal diseases have trouble hearing these good wishes. One of the chief challenges we all faced on learning we do not have long to live was the acceptance of that reality. Once we have accommodated ourselves to it, we function well. But the realization that our friends cannot also accept our time and place in life gives us a sense of isolation from them. And that can be difficult for us.

Distance, separation, isolation from the "healthy" is one of the most acute pangs for us whose days on this earth are counted in small numbers. We are not different! We are still one of you. We are not dead until we stop breathing. Every one of us, you and I, are dying from the day we're born. Don't treat us as separate. And that means not creating a fairytale scenario of what's going to happen to us, of the course of the disease that we each carry.

I have a fatal cancer. I know what I have. You know what I have. We can talk about it — in honest and forthright terms — just as we might discuss your open heart surgery, or your poison ivy, or your sprained ankle. I am no different from anyone else with any ailment. I'm living with it. I'm living.

There are some who cannot reconcile this acceptance of the inevitability of death from a current disease and the need to think positively. I can probably slow the progress of this cancer by living happily, by being upbeat. But thinking positively does not mean denial, or fiction. We reserve certain fanciful tales, like Santa Claus and the Easter Bunny and the tooth fairy, for little kids. Don't treat us like kids.

I don't mind questions like, "What's your prognosis?" or "How long have you got?" or "What type of cancer do you have?" These are the realities of my life now. They're on my mind. And they're on your mind too. We can share our thoughts. That way we're not isolated from each other.

Having written all of the above, I want to caution that this represents my feelings and the feelings of the majority of others I know who are similarly situated. But I'm not trying to tell anyone else that he or she must or should handle a fatal sickness my way. Each person has to come to this in whatever way they can. Coping with terminal illness can be very difficult and we each plot our own course.

My way is to remain as connected as possible to my friends, and that means talking about what's important to us.

Carpe diem. Enjoy today.

Dying
Was Really Living

We buried my friend Mark B. I'll miss him. His graciousness, kindness, thoughtfulness and above all his wonderful brightness and sense of humor made him a very special person. I met him only after AIDS had started its insidious ravaging of his body. But it also afforded him some of his happiest years.

Mark's first and greatest love was music. From his earliest years he doted on sitting at a keyboard — piano or organ particularly. During his teen years he was organist at a couple of churches. He spent a few years as a Jesuit, using and developing his musical talents in the service of his community. But after leaving the seminary and going into banking, the temporal and economic demands of earning a living kept him from music.

Then he found he was HIV positive. When the onset of AIDS rendered him unable to hold a job, he figured his creative days were over. Then one day he accompanied a friend to services at a church in Boston's South End, not far from Mark's apartment. The church had been for a short time without an organist and one of the staff asked Mark if he would substitute. For the first time in eight years he sat at an organ and thus began a new life. Mark's need and the church's need fit like hand and glove. The church had a new organist and Mark found his vocation again.

Mark could be found in the old cavernous church almost every day of the past few years, playing the organ. On cold winter days he kept a jacket and scarf on, while a space heater gave off a little heat behind him. Mark loved to play classical music, and the huge church reverberated to the old melodies. But some of the best sounds were those of Mark's own composition — sounds from his own heart. He was back in his element. Mark had found a bit of heaven on earth.

AIDS was not kind to Mark, but he didn't complain. Since the advent of my own terminal cancer, we found another common bond, and often compared notes on each other's progress, or lack of it. We walked together on this journey.

I had always thought that people, when told that life was approaching its end, lived on "hold" in a sort of limbo, simply waiting for death. But Mark is one of many friends I now have for whom, like the wine at the famous wedding feast at Cana, the best was saved till last. I'm not sure of all the reasons, but I think that when we're told we're not going to blow out too many more birthday candles, we're able to focus on the real priorities and screen out the unimportant and the trivial. We then can say yes to what we really want to do, and see burdensome things like work and money and grudges and sadness and worries for what they are.

I'm tempted to say that I wish I had known Mark earlier, but I had the blessing of knowing him at his best, at his happiest. For the rest of my days, whenever I enter the quiet of the Jesuit Urban Center, I'll hear the echoes of his music.

Carpe diem. Enjoy today.

Don't
Deify Doctors

"We deify these people," Mary H. was saying the other day, obviously somewhat unhappy about the proliferation of gods.

Mary H. is one of my few gurus. She is a very wise woman, kind and considerate and humorous also. I always feel a little more sage after a conversation with Mary.

We had been talking about priests, and how nuns and others must study at length to be considered qualified for counselling and spiritual direction, while the clergy are thought, by themselves and others, to have these attributes by virtue of ordination.

We had earlier been discussing medical topics, which led Mary at this point to lump doctors together with priests as classes of people that induce so many of us to suspend judgment. Otherwise intelligent people leave their cognitive facilities at the door when they enter the sanctuaries of the druids and shamans.

Doctors as a group are fairly intelligent; otherwise they never would have gotten into medical school, or out of medical school either. However, as with any other profession, there are many for whom common sense is uncommon. All doctors trained in this country are afforded a fair general grounding, then get specialized training that has to exclude many other branches of medicine. No doctor knows everything about medicine. The field is so vast today that there are areas about which any doctor knows next to nothing.

Men and women of medicine are fallible and limited, and more than likely somewhat overworked too. We do no disservice, to them or to ourselves, if we question them, if we bring the same scepticism to their diagnoses that we bring to the other technician who tells us we need a new transmission in our car. It is no insult to seek a second or a third opinion.

And there is one thing that I, the patient, know far more about than any doctor. Me. I know the pulses and rhythms of my body. I know when I am getting better and when I'm in decline. I know when a medicine is working and when it's time to go back for an alternate one.

We who have terminal ailments must bring more to the patient-doctor relationship. We have to decide for ourselves what length and quality of life we want, given, of course, the parameters of our disease. I have seen incurable cancers treated as aggressively as ones that could be conquered. All, of course, to the discomfort and distress of the patient. We, for whom medical care is, or should be, only palliative, must form clear notions of what we want from what is left to us of this life, and inform our caregivers of that. At this point I, not the doctor, am the managing partner.

We especially should decide in advance how we want to be treated at the very end, when there is no, or very little, quality of life remaining. Lacking that, we pass back to the doctor decision making that she neither wants nor should have.

Medical care, for anyone, should be a cooperative venture between the patient and the doctor, each sharing her expertise.

A*rrivederci,*
Alberto

A while ago I read the journal I kept during my sojurn in Italy. I relived the many wonderful hours, over four days, that I spent with Alberto Stefanelli and his family in Rome. He had been much on my mind anyway, because his strikingly beautiful daughter Laura had been here with me and my family.

A week after Laura was with us, I got a phone call. Alberto had died suddenly, sitting in the piazza of the little medieval Umbrian village where he was born, and where he delighted in spending his summer vacations away from the scorching heat of Rome.

Alberto and I were good friends, though we met only twice and were always separated by the inability of both of us to communicate very well in the other's language. His English was a bit better than my Italian, but that didn't matter. When we first met four years ago we were already connected by family friendships. Of the same age, we bonded instantly. Laura has been over here many times since, so we have kept in touch through her and through my relatives who travel to Italy every year.

When my wife and I went to Italy this year, we naturally let Alberto know that we were coming, and naturally, too, he and his family wanted us to spend most waking hours with them. We begged off, to leave ourselves free to wander and to avoid imposing, but we did spend parts of four days in their welcoming and happy company. Both my wife and I were worried about Alberto. While we were in Rome he returned to work after a six month hiatus because of heart problems. He did not look well. Laura told us last week that he was doing okay, but was happy to have 10 weeks off to spend in his town in the cool Umbrian hills.

I was feeling sad and somewhat depressed about the news of Alberto's death, as I poured morning coffee into a mug that reads *Carpe diem.* When the java heated the cup, the Latin words disappeared and the English translation, "Seize the Day" appeared. I reflected that this day, despite my loss, should be enjoyed.

So, while I still mourn, I will enjoy the memory of my friend. He was a big and handsome man. For many of his younger years he was a professional soccer player, and was still equally famed for his ability and enthusiasm at the dinner table. Only a bit overweight in recent years, he was quite put out over the doctor's injunction to cut down on his caloric intake. He cheated several times when we were with him in Rome. I will also enjoy the wonderful memory of our final night together, when he broke out his guitar and sang beautiful Italian songs. It was our last night in the country, and my wife wept as Alberto played "Arrivederci Roma".

We who know we're terminal have a special task at hand. We must do for others what Alberto did for me, and for so many who knew him — leave beautiful memories. (This, of course, applies to the supposedly healthy too.) Many of us can do little about the state of our health or the course of our diseases, but we can control much in our environment.

I hope that someday a few will say of me what I can say of Alberto Stefanelli today: "He was a good man. I'm grateful I knew him." Arrivederci, Alberto.

Alternative Remedies

"What do you think of alternative remedies?" a young woman, recently cured, hopefully, of breast cancer, asked me.

My answer was guarded. Certainly our western medical practitioners do not have all the answers, nor do they have all the cures. But, as the old joke goes, they are a heck of a long way ahead of whatever's in second place.

Western medicine, by which I mean the system we are used to — medication and surgery mainly — continues to learn from the "natural" medications that less sophisticated people have been using for generations, such as herb teas and poultices composed of leaves and barks. The analyses and the testing to which our drug companies, research centers and hospitals subject these remedies are wonderfully crafted and have afforded us uncounted safe medicines.

There is much that is good in patient care that our doctors have not yet learned, and here I am thinking particularly of some of the mental and physical disciplines of the East and of acupuncture in China. At the same time I am very leery of miracle "cures" that are peddled around here, and which are offered without any testing information but only with the testimony of people who have supposedly enjoyed their powers.

An old friend recently supplied me with a loose leaf folder packed with information about the power of magnets to cure a cornucopia of ailments, the theory being that all the electricity that flows through our communities disrupts our reception of the natural magnetic field of the earth — that is true — and that this is one reason for so many ailments. My friend is, not coincidentally, selling high priced mattresses and belts that have magnets implanted, to "restore" our harmony with nature. To anyone who knows anything about magnetism, this whole scheme is laughable. Elsewhere in the folder is literature proclaiming the virtues of blue-green algae. My friend is, I fear, the victim of a fraud.

Part of the pitch, which I received both in writing and orally from him, accuses our drug industry, the medical establishment and the press of a massive conspiracy to hide from us such knowledge that they already possess a cure for cancer! I tried to impress on my friend that both the press and the scientific community are today quite incapable of any such conspiracy of silence.

Somewhat inexplicably, much of the literature in the folder dwelt on the assertion that HIV does not cause AIDS! The medical community is quite aware that there are probably several other factors involved between the time someone is infected with the HIV and the time he or she starts to suffer from any of the ailments that define the AIDS stage. The thrust of these stories, of course, is to show that the medical establishment both doesn't know what it's doing and is at the same time hiding the truth from us.

The western medical establishment is far from perfect, but greed, not silence, is probably its worst sin. Thanks to the development of medical science, about 50% of cancers are today curable. The fatal cancer that dwells within my body is fairly quiet these days, affording me a period of relative good health. Had I contracted this disease 30 years ago I would have died within some months of knowing I was afflicted, mostly from pain.

Many of us who have serious and terminal ailments can get desperate. There will always be a snake oil salesman around to take advantage of our desperation.

*F*reedom to Be

I'm unsuccessfully trying to come up with an active form of the verb to be born and a passive form of the verb to die. I know we talk of "birthing", but that's the action of someone else, not the person getting born. All this came about from some reflections on death. Although we can be somewhat passive agents in the inexorable course of dying, we should be active in our lifestyle right to the end.

This cogitation came about when a nurse friend, about to participate in a workshop on humanizing death, asked for any gems of wisdom I might have. I may be in short supply of wisdom, but herewith a few thoughts anyway.

Given that we're all dying from the day we're born, I'm here discussing those last weeks or months when the ailments that ravage one's body give an indication that the coming Christmas will be one's last.

Getting back to my grammar question about active and passive, permit a dying person have as great a role in her process as she wants. Do not deny her freedom. Already the disease has robbed her of much independence, particularly the liberty of growing older. Don't further shackle her. So what if she wants to eat or drink something that's "bad" for her, or to smoke. Or she wants to engage in "dangerous" activity. So her life might be shortened by another few days. Big deal. It's the quality, not the number of days, that matters.

Listen to her. Give her the opportunity to talk. She may want to talk about her impending death. Give her the chance to do so. That might be more than you can handle. Then bring in someone, a hospice worker, a clergyman perhaps, who can afford her the opportunity to unburden herself. There may be old wounds that she wants to heal. Give her the chance. Listen.

Does she have any unfinished business? Things she must do to feel free to die? Are there unfulfilled ambitions that can still be achieved. Again, listen to her.

Speaking of clergymen, don't expect them or doctors to be able to handle death any better than the rest of us. Many of them can't talk about it either, so know who you're bringing in.

Doctors. Yes, doctors. Many are quite inept in handling the human aspects of dying. They're trained to heal, and some of them see a death as their failure. I see a lot of dying people now, and so often I'm appalled at the vigorous treatment they're undergoing when there can be absolutely no benefit. A dying person can sometimes be made more comfortable by treatments like radiation, but some doctors just don't know when to stop.

Pain is an adjunct of many deaths, particularly for those of us with cancer. Morphine and other anesthetics alleviate that pain. Often doctors are afraid to order large enough doses, because it can be a shot of morphine that finally causes a person *in extremis* to stop breathing. I've even heard doctors quoted as saying they don't want to addict the patient!

Don't start the wake and funeral before the person is dead. Enjoy her company now. Make her environment a happy place. If she wants company, make sure people come to see her. If she wants to party, have parties. Take her to parties. Yes, I know that others may be uncomfortable in her presence. They'll get over it.

And finally, surround her with love. Make sure she sees and hears from those who are closest to her. Dying is a lonely experience, and we have to do it by ourselves, but we can be mightily helped by knowing we're appreciated. There are no words that can assist the process more than, "I love you, darling."

Carpe diem. Enjoy today. And make sure she does.

Carpe Diem

From the beginning of this book, I've been using the expression *Carpe diem*. The expression is neither mine nor Robin Williams', who used it repeatedly and pointedly in *The Dead Poets Society,* a fine movie.

The words come from a work of the noted Roman poet of two millennia ago, Quintus Horatius Flaccus, whom we call Horace. In the eleventh ode of book one, he used the words *Carpe diem*, literally, "seize the day," or better, "enjoy today." For many years the words *Carpe diem* have been current in English. I've known many people virginal of Latin who use them. So, 'tis time. Here is the whole of Horace's poem.

Tu ne quaesieris — scire nefas — quem mihi, quem tibi finem di dederint, Leuconoe, nec Babylonios temptaris numeros. ut melius, quicquid erit, pati! seu plures hiemes, seu tribuit Iuppiter ultimam, quae nunc oppositis debilitat pumicibus mare Tyrrhenum. sapias, vina liques, et spatio brevi spem longam reseces. dum loquimur, fugerit invida aetas; carpe diem, quam minumum credula postero.

It is virtually impossible to translate poetry from one language to another. But here is my own version, rendered as prose.

Don't ask — it's forbidden to know — Leuconoe, what ending the gods will give you or me. So don't try the Babylonian numbers. Better to endure whatever will be, whether Jupiter allows us many winters or is giving us the last one which is now wearing out the Tyrrhenian Sea on the barrier cliffs. Be wise, strain your wine, and quickly cut short your long range hopes. While we speak, jealous time flees. Enjoy today. Put as little trust as possible into tomorrow.

And the explanation:

I don't know who Leuconoe is. He might have been a buddy of Horace, or it might be a made up name to fit the metre. That's still done, you know. Steven Foster's famous Swanee River got its inspiration from the Suwannee River, but the extra syllable got in the way.

The Babylonian numbers referred to throws of the dice or other calculations of the astrologers from the East. Babylon was close to where Baghdad is now, and at the moment we don't trust any numbers or information coming from there, either.

"Strain your wine" seems to be a suggestion to take care of simple household tasks.

So there it is. Not bad advice from an old pagan. Horace was a poet of simple things, of enjoyment of life, nature, love, drinking, youth, home, leisure. Most of us could learn a lot from him. He lived, as we do, in a very tumultuous time but insisted on enjoying and praising the simple pleasures.

So whether you are in good health or ill, whether you are young or old or somewhere in between, whether you expect this to be your last winter or plan on dozens more, enjoy today.

Carpe diem!